Whistleblowing in the
Health Service

Whistleblowing in the Health Service

Accountability, Law and Professional Practice

Edited by

Geoffrey Hunt

Director
European Centre for Professional Ethics
University of East London
London
and
National Coordinator, Freedom to Care

Edward Arnold
A member of the Hodder Headline Group
LONDON MELBOURNE AUCKLAND

First published in Great Britain 1995 by Edward Arnold,
a division of Hodder-Headline PLC, 338 Euston Road, London NW1 3BH

British Library Cataloguing in Publication Data

A catalogue record for this book is available from the British Library

ISBN 0 340 59234 6

1   2   3   4   5   95   96   97   98   99

Typeset in 10/11pt Times by Phoenix Photosetting, Chatham, Kent.
Printed and bound in Great Britain by J. W. Arrowsmith Ltd, Bristol.

Contents

Notes on the contributors

Alan Hannah is a partner in Brachers Solicitors, Chancery Lane, London and previously a part time Industrial Tribunal chairman.

Toby Harris is the Director of the Association of Community Health Councils, London.

Geoffrey Hunt is the Director of the European Centre for Professional Ethics, University of East London, London and the National Coordinator of Freedom to Care. He is the editor of *Ethical Issues in Nursing*, Routledge, 1994 and (with Paul Wainwright) *Expanding the Role of the Nurse*, Blackwell Scientific, 1994.

Diane Longley lectures in the Centre for Socio-Legal Studies, Sheffield University and is the author of *Public Law & Health Service Accountability*, Open University Press, 1993.

Jean McHale lectures in the Law Faculty, University of Manchester and is the author of *Medical Confidentiality & Legal Privilege*, Routledge, 1993.

Jean Orr is Professor in the School of Nursing Studies, Queen's University of Belfast, is a member of the United Kingdom Central Council for Nursing, Midwifery and Health Visiting and the editor (with Karen Luker) of *Health Visiting*, Blackwell Scientific, 1985.

David Pilgrim is a Senior Research Fellow in the Health and Community Care Research Unit, University of Liverpool and is the editor (with A. Rogers) of *A Sociology of Mental Health and Illness*, Open University Press, 1993.

Ray Rowden is the Director of the Institute of Health Services Management, London.

Barbara Shailer is Principal Lecturer in the Department of Nursing and Health Studies, Middlesex University, Enfield, Middlesex.

Meg Stacey is Professor Emeritus in Sociology, Warwick University and is the author of *Regulating British Medicine*, Wiley, 1992.

Andrew Wall is Senior Fellow, Health Services Management Centre, School of Public Policy, University of Birmingham and is the author of *Ethics and the Health Services Manager*, King's Fund, 1989. He was for 18 years the District General Manager, Bath District Health Authority.

Marlene Winfield is a trustee of the charity and legal advice centre, Public Concern at Work, London and the author of *Minding Your Own Business: Self-Regulation and Whistleblowing in British Companies*, Social Audit, London, 1990.

Foreword

I have spent most of my professional life at the Bar in the field of employment law. I noticed early on that our National Health Service seemed to spend inordinate time and resources in displaying in the Industrial Tribunals, in which I used frequently to appear, a standard and style of industrial relations which were quite unique in their inept insensitivity and arrogant incompetence.

Multinational corporations, nationalised industries, civil service departments, local authorities, manufacturing companies, service industries, retail outlets, media consortia, even 'cowboy' builders – no class of employer seemed as impoverished in terms of 'human resource management' as the various health authorities I observed in the Tribunals.

I often wondered why this should be. I assumed that it was statistical aberration that dropped briefs against such consistently inadequate employers on to my desk. This book proves I was wrong. What I observed was not merely chance but a manifestation of structural defects far more profound and at much higher level than the personality of managers.

This first class analysis of whistleblowing in the health service sets out the many factors which underlie the fact that so many have been punished for daring to raise 'at least one concern about some important issues of policy, practice or standards' in the hope of improving those things. The book deals with the underlying themes of accountability and autonomy, of confidentiality and freedom of speech. It deals with the tension between the standards established by the professional bodies and the dictates of the contract of employment.

The book will be of immense value to all who work in the NHS at all levels. It will also be of value to lawyers and other concerned outsiders. In the last couple of years I represented Dr Helen Zeitlin, the consultant haematologist who was purportedly dismissed on the alleged ground of redundancy, having dared to raise publicly her fears about shortage of nurses on her wards. I also represented Mr Graham Pink, the nurse who was dismissed for complaining of the shortage of nurses on his wards. Both, happily, were vindicated, but the fact that they felt that they had to go outside the service to raise their points and the fact that they were in consequence punished, demonstrates the need for this book to raise the profile of this problem.

The authors do not just raise the issue of whistleblowing, they also point ways forward. The problems are plainly remediable, and it is to be hoped that the Secretary of State and Government will take note of this book. For it is at that level that the initiative for change needs to come. Only then will there be a resolution of the paradox whereby staff are required to provide the highest level of care to their patients and are themselves denied a basic level of justice.

John Hendy QC

Preface

My concern about the travails of conscientious employees has its origins in my experiences as an academic at the University College of Swansea. In 1989 Anne Maclean and I officially raised concerns with our line managers about standards on a Masters Degree in the Philosophy of Health Care. Prior to that moment we had believed that our suggestions and constructive criticism would eventually be received and acted upon in a cooperative spirit. I had not the least inkling of the furore that would build up over the next three years because of the uncompromising nature of the institution in which I was an employee. I could not have foreseen that I would resign in the summer of 1990, that Anne would be pressured into signing a severance contract which completely silenced her, and that two other colleagues would be suspended for supporting us. It would have been unimaginable that three internal inquiries and two public inquiries (one headed by Sir Peter Swinnerton-Dyer and the other by Sir Michael Davies) would be necessary to address our plain and simple concerns. Without the dogged and wily perseverance of Mike Cohen and Colwyn Williamson, both suspended for over two years on full pay, I have no doubt whatsoever that we four would have been silenced, academic malpractice would have continued and standards would have deteriorated. Thanks to Cohen and Williamson here was a lesson for all – for the institution and for The Swansea Four.

When the four of us were given Freedom of Information Awards in January 1994 a journalist asked me whether I felt it had all been worth it. I am sure I can speak for the four of us in saying of course it has been worth it. Changes have taken place at the University College of Swansea, university managers and staff all over the country have taken heed, and the labour pains of The Swansea Four have given birth to two organisations dedicated to assisting other conscientious employees.

I moved to Queen Charlotte's College of Healthcare Studies, based at the Hammersmith Hospital, where I was given the task of creating and running a centre for studying problems of ethics and accountability in nursing, midwifery and health visiting. Grateful as I was for this opportunity, it proved to be unsustainable. At the end of October 1992 I circulated a leaflet announcing the launch, at the House of Commons, of Freedom to Care – a non-party network of public sector 'whistleblowers' and their supporters. Four days later, by a most remarkable coincidence, I was told that I was being made redundant – the only member of staff who was dispensable. It appeared that there was a 'problem with overspend' and that 'ethics is a luxury'. My life as the

NHS's first, and almost certainly last, social philosopher was over after only two and a half years. Fortunately, the University of East London was able to provide me with a new home – from which I was able to edit this book.

Meanwhile, the other three members of The Swansea Four have set up the Council for Academic Freedom and Academic Standards (CAFAS), with aims similar to Freedom to Care, and concentrating on the further and higher education sector. Both organisations continue to grow.

I am grateful to many members of Freedom to Care for their ideas and encouragement in writing my sections of this book. But I must emphasize that this is not a publication of Freedom to Care and that it would be quite wrong to associate any particular contributor with Freedom to Care or its aims and activities.

I thank the Confederation of Health Service Employees (now part of UNISON) for a grant to the European Centre for Professional Ethics, University of East London, to cover the expenses involved in travelling all over England to interview the subjects in the research project published in Chapter one. Marlene Winfield and Ann Kennedy made helpful suggestions in designing the project.

I very much appreciate the support given to me by the University of East London, and especially Professor John Neville and Ms Linda Hanford.

The United Kingdom Central Council for Nursing, Midwifery and Health Visiting kindly gave permission to reproduce sections from the Registrar's Letter 37 (14 Dec 1992), 'Standards for Incorporation into Contracts for Hospital and Community Health care Services' in Chapter 4.

I would be pleased to receive comments and criticisms about this book from individuals and organisations, as well as inquiries about Freedom to Care. The address is PO Box 125, West Molesey, Surrey, KT8 1YE.

Geoffrey Hunt

Introduction: Whistleblowing and the breakdown of accountability

Geoffrey Hunt

The whistleblower in everyone

In every general social crisis the clear simplicity of the Manichaean scheme of things is very appealing and always takes hold. It is also very useful to the status quo: the system is really quite sound, but there are people who abuse it, 'bad apples'. Sir John May's five-year, £2 million inquiry into the Guildford Four jailing uncovered some bad apples, and since there will always be that type there really is no point in saying who they are. There are, of course, the 'good apples', the great and good Establishment figures who head public inquiries and put everything right again. Recently, a peculiar and fascinating hybrid has started to make its appearance, that is the whistleblower – half trouble-maker, half-hero.

The plot is exceedingly simple. The whistleblower points out the bad apples, the bad apples fight back, the whistleblower is expelled from the applecart. There are two conclusions. The whistleblower is ruined, and we bystanders look on wringing our hands. The good apples intervene, the balance of the applecart is restored, and the bystanders applaud.

Of course, these are all creatures of our own imagination. The most interesting of them are not those on the applecart. The bystander is central to the real plot, for without him or her the other three would have no life at all. To understand our social crisis it is the bystander who needs examination. To this end it would have been preferable to have produced a collection of essays about bystanders, but it is hardly likely that this would have attracted much attention at the present time. All eyes are on the applecart – that is the problem. As Bertolt Brecht knew, it takes some time and effort to destroy the theatrical illusion so as to prevent the audience becoming emotionally involved in the play and examining themselves. It is hoped that these reflections will make a small, if undoubtedly rather jumbled, beginning in enabling us all to view the subject matter with some objectivity and insight. We have to start questioning our own social attitudes and perceptions, if we are to gain any grasp of the systemic crisis to which, and of which, we are subject.

After the May Inquiry the 'bad apple' theory will no doubt begin to lose credence in every quarter. Now that we face almost weekly failures and scandals in our public life, it is becoming clearer that what is at stake is the very legitimacy of the systems that we have taken for granted for several decades. Dramatic failures in the executive arm of government, the judicial system, the legislature, the police, the civil service and local government, the penal system, banking and insurance, the universities, and health and social welfare point to a fundamental democratic deficit and a crisis of legitimation.

'Whistleblowing' belongs to the realm of psychopathological symptoms. The underlying condition is dangerous, namely a deep schism in our social life, in particular the isolation of our public institutions and private corporations, and their goals and methods, from the common welfare of citizens. There is a widening gulf between what we know as individuals to be right and good and the near impossibility of living by this knowledge in the workplace. Whistleblowing occurs at the unsettling intersection of an increasingly generalised allegiance to personal autonomy, and civil and human rights, and the decreasing public accountability of our institutions. All of us are experiencing less and less confidence in paternalistic experts, politicians, mandarins and managers at the very moment we are experiencing a loss of a voice, of control, of meaning in the work we do – if we are lucky enough to work. In the whistleblower there is projected that small piece of all of us, the part that says 'Whatever the Institution tells me, I know I'm right and it is wrong'. Meanwhile, the bystander stays in control as there is too much to lose.

It follows that whistleblowers personally have nothing in common. What they have in common is that they have blown the whistle, and it is precisely in this, like the deeds and fate of the Tolpuddle Martyrs perhaps, that we could find a new way of understanding ourselves and our social predicament.

Conscientious employees who persevere, against the resistance of management, to raise a workplace concern in the public interest probably existed long before they came to be regarded as whistleblowers. But pre-modern whistleblowers were only such in the same way in which, say, the cowrie shells of some traditional African societies were money. The shells come to be seen as a form of money only when a certain highly developed form of exchange dominates and can provide us with such a perspective – a perspective from which a 'history of money' could be written. So it is that when the autonomous rights-bearing individual comes to dominate as a form of being-in-society that the whistleblower emerges. As money appears against a backdrop of commodity production, so whistleblowing emerges against the backdrop of closed, unresponsive and bureaucratic institutions of employment. Andrei

Sakharov and the other dissidents of the old Soviet system might now figure in a history of whistleblowing, but their scenario was not the workplace. In the UK the history of whistleblowing properly begins with the health and social services.

The whistleblower's experience

Whistleblowing surfaced in the UK health service in an atmosphere of apprehension and anxiety. Economic recession and public expenditure cuts, combined with the imposition of commercial-style management on the National Health Service, have threatened standards of care, disempowered health care professionals and almost certainly created new conditions for negligence and abuse, and new opportunities for fraud and corruption. Three recent cases in particular have become icons of professional dissidence: Graham Pink, a charge nurse, who went public over standards of care on a ward in a Stockport hospital, and was dismissed (*The Guardian*, 1990); Helen Zeitlin, a doctor who expressed concern about a nursing shortage in her Redditch hospital and was made redundant (*The Guardian*, 1992a); and Chris Chapman, principal biochemist working for Leeds General Infirmary and Leeds University, made redundant following his claim that scientific fraud was taking place under commercial pressures (*Laboratory Practice*, 1992). Since then the situation hardly appears to have improved. The whistleblowing has continued, despite a worsening mood of fear, following on from closures and mass redundancies, gagging clauses in contracts of employment (*The Independent on Sunday*, 1991; *The Guardian*, 1992b) and, most recently, the bugging of a consultant's office by the Luton and Dunstable Hospital Trust chief executive (*The Guardian*, 1994).

A survey conducted by the union, Manufacturing Science Finance (MSF), and published in February 1993, showed that fear of losing their jobs was keeping NHS staff from talking to the media about malpractice and poor standards. That survey of over 50 media health correspondents showed that in the two years since the NHS reforms were introduced staff have increasingly become too frightened to speak out publicly on standards of patient care, fraud and misconduct in the health service. MSF says:

> Regional health correspondents, who have been the traditional mouthpiece for exposing malpractice at local level, expressed the most concern. Many said that stories on the health service had begun to dry up since the reforms and gagging clauses had come into effect (MSF, 1993).

Journalists also claimed it was increasingly difficult to gain access to information about the public services.

The escalation of institutional intimidation mirrors the situation of the individual whistleblower. Management often deals with staff concerns in a sensitive, efficient and fair manner. Often they do not and sometimes, one suspects, they cannot. In the worst scenario, events unfold something like this. The conscientious employee raises a concern and fails to have it addressed. Instead of letting it go the employee takes the concern one stage further, and then another. The tension winds up a notch at a time. The authorities are still unresponsive, believing perhaps that the problem will fade away. The stakes become higher, for both employee and employer, neither wishing to lose face. The complainant becomes more indignant, the authorities are now determined to shut him or her up, and even more resolute when they see that their failure to act on the concern and their intimidation of the complainant may be exposed. There is now a confrontation, the authorities have their reputation to lose, the complainant his or her job. At any stage the complainant may withdraw. If they persevere, they may be dismissed. The authorities calculate that an industrial tribunal may go in their favour, and if it does not then they will settle with a large payment at the last moment and let their public relations officer make the best of it. At least they will have rid themselves of the trouble-maker.

The UK survey reported in Chapter 1 provides a more detailed outline of how this escalation takes place. It follows on a recent survey of 35 whistleblowers in Australia who had exposed corruption or danger to the public. The Australian questionnaire survey was carried out among whistleblowers who contacted Whistleblowers Australia (founded July 1991), an organisation very similar to Freedom to Care in the UK. The account of the methods employed by conscientious employees to have their complaints addressed, and their consequent experiences, tally closely with the experiences of whistleblowers in touch with the UK organisation. The Australian report says:

> All subjects had started by making a complaint internally, through what they considered were the proper channels. Three had not made a complaint but submitted a report during the normal course of their duties. Three subjects had not progressed beyond making an internal complaint. The remaining 32 had subsequently complained to some official external body – for example, ombudsmen, members of parliament, their union, the Independent Commission Against Corruption, the auditor general. . . . Only 17 subjects had approached the media and then only after exhausting internal and external avenues.
>
> Fifty external bodies were mentioned, covering several states, so the numbers for each were small. Only three were rated as helpful by more than one person. Unions scored two helpful ratings but also six harmful, seven neither helpful nor harmful, and one hopeless. Only six bodies scored any helpful mentions, while there were 22 harmful and 51 neither helpful nor harmful mentions.
>
> The problem complained of continued unchanged or increased in 25 cases, decreased in four, and was unknown in the remaining six. No action had

been taken against those responsible or they had been promoted in 30 cases, and in five cases those responsible had received minor disciplinary action. In only one case were all those responsible disciplined and none promoted.

(Lennane, 1993)

The report remarks on the close similarities in the kind of treatment the institution meted out to the complainants. Any UK whistleblower who reads this report may experience that mixed feeling of dismay at so much suffering like their own and relief that they are not after all alone. The Report states at one point, 'Some techniques, such as putting the whistleblower in a bare office with no telephone, seem also diagnostic'. In the UK whistleblowers Mike Cohen and Colwyn Williamson at University College Swansea (see Preface) were moved out of their Philosophy Department offices into shabby rooms in the Maintenance Department without telephones.

The report closes with advice for doctors caring for whistleblowers. This is good advice, but something about the entire approach adopted in the report is discomfiting. The message which this study appears to be giving to conscientious employees, whatever the intention, is this: if you are thinking of making a complaint, however legitimate, however appalling the situation about which you wish to complain, then you must expect to be made sick, sacked, financially ruined and at the end of the day your complaint will almost certainly not have been addressed.

Multi-level breakdown

The UK survey discussed in Chapter 1 also indicates how whistleblowing is a failure at several levels. It is symptomatic of a multi-layered breakdown in accountability. Some cases strongly suggest a pervasive reluctance within the health (and social) services to respect due process and deal with matters in a fair and cooperative spirit. One would not expect a microbiologist employed by the NHS to have to struggle through the courts for 10 years finally to arrive at the European Court of Human Rights to obtain justice – and yet this is what happened to Dr Royce Darnell (*The Whistle* 2, 1993, p. 5).

Dr Darnell, one-time head of Derby Royal Infirmary's microbiology laboratory, was suspended in 1982 by his employer for alleged non-compliance with management procedures. After a local inquiry he was dismissed in 1984 by Trent Regional Health Authority. He appealed to the Secretary of State and won. This was ignored by the Department of Health and Social Security administrators. He went to the courts for a judicial review to order his re-employment. He won that too. Again this was ignored, and his dismissal confirmed. Then followed a succession of court applications to no avail. Finally, after years of struggle, Dr Darnell took his case to the European Court of Human Rights. The

Commissioners first heard his case and were unanimous in deciding that his human rights had been violated. They recommended a settlement. This proved impossible due to the intransigence of the NHS which refused to release a key document that was at the heart of the matter. The case was heard by the full Court of Human Rights. At the Court in April 1993 the UK representatives finally admitted that Dr Darnell's civil rights had been violated. The UK Government has now offered to pay all of Dr Darnell's costs.

Another case shows how ethical questions may be raised about management and administration, employment law, the working of industrial tribunals, charities and self-regulation. A manager concerned about the care of his clients felt he was put in an ethically untenable position (*The Whistle* 3, 1993, p. 5). Ron Thomson worked as General Manager/Company Secretary of a charity running a number of care homes for people with learning difficulties – until February 1992, when he resigned. For over a year he had been complaining about the quality of care provided to residents by staff employed by the local health authority but working under contract to the charity. He also reported to his board of directors that, in his opinion, several abuses of the law were occurring within the Registered Care Homes. As the registered Person in Control he could have personally been prosecuted and banned from any involvement in any registered care.

An internal group was established to try to resolve the problems but it appeared to Thomson to be whitewashing the care contractors (the group's chairperson was the Chief Executive of the care agency concerned). After allegedly being instructed to destroy a report which he had written giving details of financial and physical abuse of residents as well as several other breaches of the Registered Homes Act, Thomson believed he had no option but to resign. Thomson lost the Industrial Tribunal hearing at which he claimed constructive dismissal. Ron Thomson writes:

> Is it acceptable for an employer to expect employees to do something they consider to be unprofessional, bad practice, immoral or illegal? The law is, in practice at least, rather unclear about it. Industrial tribunals have, in the past, often looked solely at aspects of employment law. They have ignored other issues such as professional body regulations and codes of practice. They have even disregarded actions the employee has had to take (e.g. resignation) to protect themselves from potential prosecution in the courts. There have been a number of cases of apparent injustice at industrial tribunals arising where employees have taken the step of refusing to comply with instructions which they considered to be wrong, or even illegal. However, many of these people were not supported by tribunal decisions because they had on previous occasions carried out those same instructions. It seems that if you carry out an employer's instruction once you are almost legally bound to continue doing it for ever – even if you only become aware of the fact it is illegal or bad practice later.

(*The Whistle* 3, 1993, p. 5)

The breakdown of accountability may, as we well know from recent government failures, reach up to Members of Parliament, government departments and Secretaries of State.

In one recent case, a black health visitor, Desmond Smith, who blew the whistle on racial abuse sent a dossier from his disciplinary hearing to his Member of Parliament for advice (*The Whistle* **2**, 1993, p. 3). Instead of helping his constituent, the MP sent the dossier back to the very managers with whom Smith was in dispute. These managers consequently dropped the original charges and sacked him for breach of confidentiality instead. The regulatory body (in this case the English National Board) found Smith had no case to answer. When the case reached an Industrial Tribunal the authority understood its mistake, acknowledged unfair dismissal, and Smith was awarded a record sum of £27 000. No action was subsequently taken against the managers.

One may wonder how this MP understood his accountability to the public. Furthermore, it is an example of how close we are to allowing infringements of a fundamental democratic right and privilege – to speak to one's MP at any time about any matter in confidence. (It may well be that this MP was the one who breached confidentiality.) Section 27 of the NHS Management Executive's 'Guidance for Staff on Relations with the Public and the Media' appeared to override this right (NHSME, 1993). The most charitable view is that the section was drafted awkwardly. In any case, the Secretary of State had to give a public assurance that the constitutional right was being respected. In a House of Commons Health Committee debate on this very matter Mrs Bottomley said 'I can conceive of no circumstances where simply speaking to the MP was the cause of disciplinary proceedings' (*The Whistle* **4**, 1994, p. 8). Freedom to Care wrote to Mrs Bottomley to draw her attention to the Desmond Smith case, only to receive the unhelpful reply from an NHS Executive officer that 'Mr Smith was dismissed for breaching patient confidentiality and not for raising a concern with a Member of Parliament' (NHS Executive letter, 1994). What this ignores is that Smith supposedly breached confidentiality in writing (with a dossier of supporting evidence) to his MP, and not in any other act of his.

The Smith case, then, raises questions about disciplinary procedures, the law relating to confidentiality, constitutional rights, employment law, the behaviour of MPs, and the power of the regulatory bodies for the professions.

Separation of powers

One has only to examine any whistleblowing case in detail to unravel a complex web of problems with ramifications for several different institutional systems. A whistleblowing case is rarely about one 'deaf' manager. Anyone who deals with a large number of these cases is likely to grow very uneasy about our current institutional frameworks and assumptions. Something is pervasively wrong, but what? I think a useful approach to the problem is the traditional concept of 'separation of powers'. So often it appears that powers which should be separate, or indeed were separate at one time, are not. This approach at least suggests certain remedies (see my Conclusion).

There is a already a national debate about quangos (quasi-autonomous non-governmental organisations) and the way in which the probity that might be expected from them is endangered by a blurring or duplication of roles and responsibilities. It should be obvious enough that someone who has, for example, a monitoring role on behalf of the public welfare should not at the same time have commercial interests which could compromise the independence and impartiality of that role. Yet this kind of failure to separate powers is now endemic, resulting in a kind of political mushiness which is characteristic of totalitarianism.

In Chapter 2 Andrew Wall asks if recent governments have confused 'governing' with 'managing'. Such a confusion, he says, leads to 'centralised decision-making and incurring the frustration of managers and sometimes their contempt for politicians' (p. 23). Civil servants protecting a minister against embarrassing questions in parliament may seek 'information' from NHS managers, and although managers should not unreasonably withhold information the civil servants should not 'use their authority in a threatening manner'. Wall speaks of 'patronage' and 'informal but powerful influences' and says this 'threatens the safeguarding of standards' (p. 24).

Health authorities, in their new role as purchasers, should be aware of community needs and act as the advocates of the community. But how is this possible when the community has in most cases little or no voice on the authority, a body which is in any case unelected? It would appear that a health authority simply arrogates to itself the role of community voice, so that the managerial power of purchasers is not separated from and subordinated to patients and community. Wall suggests that if a health authority does happen to listen to, and defend the interests of, the community it serves it may be accused by government of 'playing politics' (p. 25). In truth civil servants who use non-statutory means to enforce implementation are playing politics.

The failure of many health authorities to assist the whistleblower by impartially investigating the concerns raised points to a reluctance or an inability to act as advocates of the community. In most cases they do not, for example, seem to work particularly closely with community health councils (CHCs). As Toby Harris points out in Chapter 5, CHCs were set up in part as a means of separating management interests from patient and community interests, and avoiding conflicts between the two (p. 69). But the reforms have weakened the CHC role.

Problems with the separation of powers appear in several guises in the new managed market, especially in the sphere of contracting and purchasing. Whistleblowing can arise in the vacuum left by substituting clinical autonomy and judgement with an unreasonable degree of managerial *specification*. Purchasers and their consultants and the suppliers are often intimately connected. The contractual relationship, says Wall, 'tends to be concerned primarily with what gets done rather than how'. This creates plenty of space for concerns about standards which the new system cannot address. We really have to ask how the specification is arrived at in the first place, how it is understood, and how it relates to what patients and nurses would regard as adequate standards.

Whistleblowing occurred in the health service in the 1960s and 1970s, especially in the context of special hospitals and care of the mentally ill. What, therefore, is the link between recent reforms and public expenditure cuts and whistleblowing? David Pilgrim points out in Chapter 6 that many factors can influence the quality of practice, including institutional isolation and staff prejudices. The Ashworth special hospital scandal (DoH, 1992) had little to do with resource shortage, while the Graham Pink case appears to have had everything to do with it. However, the recent attempt to impose a market ideology has given whistleblowing a new dimension and a certain inevitability. The market world of consumers expressing their choices by making purchases – in which illness, disease, disability and infirmity are market opportunities and health care is a commodity – flattens all roles into buying and selling. This radically undermines a welfare system supported by an ethic of public service, democratic representation and the separation of powers. Health care professionals can no longer expect clinical judgement to take precedence, because market demand and supply intrude more or less directly into clinical judgement.

Health care professionals who always took the service ethic and clinical autonomy for granted now find that they have to speak out to defend it in the face of forces which appear to have little to do with any ethic whatsoever. Thus, one fundamental question is whether it is at all acceptable to allow the market to test health care options. Even the New Right ideologists may find this difficult to answer. As Wall puts it, 'as the failure of a part of the health service may be beyond what is politically tolerable, the discipline of the market is considerably compromised' (p. 26). That is, poorly made shoes wear out and people soon learn not to buy them, so that the manufacturer has to improve or face bankruptcy. Ought we allow this to apply with treatment and care of the sick and disabled? Whistleblowing is certainly about standards, but its basic premise is the service ethic, and that is why so many whistleblowers feel so strongly – their impulse is a moral one.

Confidentiality

The powerful forces now at work in the health service are creating dislocations not only in organisation but in the very language and concepts of care. The very notion of confidentiality, understood in the context of professional ethics, is being challenged by a notion of confidentiality which comes from quite a different environment – the environment of business.

In the business arena confidentiality would appear to rest on proprietary rights and the protection of information vital to the profit and success of a business. The one profession which is more familiar with this sense of 'confidentiality' is perhaps that of accountancy and financial auditing. There the law and professional practice seem to be at one in prohibiting disclosure of information gained in the performance of an audit. (Recently, the BBC had difficulties in transmitting a *Panorama* programme about alleged corruption in Westminster City Council because of section 30 of the 1982 Local Government Act, which apparently protects witnesses who have given evidence to a district auditor.) It is, however, alien to health care in the UK.

I think we may be seeing in some controversies a confusion of confidentiality taken from professional ethics, with the purpose of protecting patients and respecting their autonomy, with commercial confidentiality and trade secrecy taken from the context of business, with the purpose of protecting competitiveness and profits.

Although the law does impinge on matters of confidentiality and disclosure most professionals do not put the emphasis on this. Professional health carers have not (at least not until recently) conceived confidentiality in the context of civil law or the law of contract. Most health care professionals (especially doctors) regard the principle of confidentiality as one which they have themselves developed along with the evolution of their practice, and it precedes the current legal concept. Professional codes of conduct for doctors, nurses and others all enshrine an explicit clause about respecting patient confidentiality. For doctors this goes back to the Hippocratic Oath of the 5th century BC.

Indeed, confidentiality arises intrinsically from the professional relationship and is a concept in professional conduct and ethics, and is not something imposed on the professions from the outside. It is seen as a matter of keeping private the information which is divulged by individuals in their specific capacity as patients or clients. The professional only has that information because the individual has entered into a narrowly-defined relationship for the purpose of receiving expert assistance. The professional only has that information *qua* professional, and has no right to dispose of it except in so far as it plays a part in discharging that duty of assistance.

This implies something else of great importance: the interests of the client are paramount. This is stated explicitly, for example, in the nurses' code of conduct (UKCC, 1989, secs. H1, H2). If the professional relationship rests on expert help then the rationale for the relationship is the need of the individual who seeks help. The relationship has no foundation, no justification except for the need or perceived need of the individual, who in perceiving his need as something amenable to expert help is thereby defining himself as a client, as a patient (i.e. as someone for whom or to whom something may be done by someone who has special knowledge). The interests of the professional, or indeed of management or of the institution, may also be served but not independently of the interests of clients, present and future.

Thus the general purpose of *professional* confidentiality is not to protect the professional, nor is it to protect management or the health care institution. This is the general supposition against which we may allow the possibility of exceptional situations, in which the protection of the professional, the management or the institution is demonstrably a means (perhaps rather indirect) of protecting clients.

The principle of confidentiality is never, in professional ethics, framed in absolute terms. That is, professionals are not expected to respect confidentiality under all circumstances. While there is a presupposition in favour of confidentiality the professional nearly always has to balance harms and benefits.

It is enlightening to ask what kind of criteria are used in establishing the proper balance. It might be thought that one has to balance, for example, administrative or managerial considerations against ethical considerations of harm. Thus an administrator might say, 'Perhaps we ought to disclose this information, but it will cost us some money to do so, so we won't'. Financial cost is not on the face of it an ethical consideration and should not go into the balance. What goes into the balance should all be ethical considerations. Thus, for example, a doctor may have to weigh up the harm to his patient who suffers from a mental illness of disclosing certain information to a relative about the illness against the benefits for the patient of such disclosure. Here the doctor is weighing a moral harm against a moral good.

Abuse of the principle

The principle of confidentiality residing in the professional context may be, and I believe is being, abused (or, more charitably, misunderstood) in some quarters. I have already referred to the case of Desmond Smith, and the research reported in Chapter 1 shows how often 'breach of confidentiality' is used to expel the whistleblower.

Clauses which gag employees are widespread in contracts of employment. More worrying perhaps are severance contracts which gag the departing member of staff. Two whistleblowers in higher education – at University College of Swansea and Bournemouth University – have admitted to signing such severance contracts (*The Whistle* 3, 1993, p. 6), but although this is happening in the health service too it has not yet received publicity.

Michael Douglas (1994), a London barrister, pointed out at a recent seminar on 'Confidentiality or Gagging, Where is the Dividing Line?', organised by the European Centre for Professional Ethics, University of East London and Brachers Solicitors, that many current confidentiality clauses in employment contracts are too broad. Consider clauses such as: 'I undertake to treat as confidential all information derived from or obtained during or after my employment at X Hospital. I understand that failure to do so may result in disciplinary action which may result in dismissal'. Michael Douglas observed:

> This example, taken from an actual contract, shows the problems which can arise in the drafting of such obligations. Strictly construed the above term would place an employee in breach of her contract if she divulged the fact that the coffee vending machine very often gave her white coffee when she pressed the black coffee button.... The Court would look at such a term and, whilst acknowledging that parties are free to agree whatever restrictions they wish, would conclude that it was either 1) meaningless, because it is inherently absurd or contradictory to consider the sort of information described as 'confidential' or 2) in restraint of trade by fettering to a far greater extent than the employer's interests could conceivably justify, an employee's basic right to use knowledge and experience gained in the course of employment as part of his skill and know-how.... Many of the confidentiality provisions contained in contracts are so vague and badly drawn that they would not withstand close judicial scrutiny. As a general rule a 'catch all' clause will be void.
>
> (Douglas, 1994)

In Chapter 11 Alan Hannah reviews the question of confidentiality and the public interest in relation to the existing employment law. While it would appear to be just that an employer should have protection from the unscrupulous employee who wishes to take trade secrets and set up business or sell them to another, the question arises how far this protection should properly be taken.

Hannah distinguishes between information which is confidential because it rests on respect for patients and the private lives of staff (e.g. matters in personnel files) and information about the general economic and managerial aspects of a health care unit which might embarrass managers but which is of doubtful confidentiality in a body serving the public (p. 146).

Professional self-regulation

Raising the issue of confidentiality and gagging in the context of professional ethics is important because it is quite possible that professional self-regulation will come under threat just as the autonomy of the health care professional is under threat.

It is true that the professions have themselves sometimes been guilty of overstretching or even abusing the principle of confidentiality. The possibility is inherent in the professional relationship. This is because confidentiality is at once a protection of the client and a protection of the professional, for unless the client feels protected the professional role itself is undermined. That is, while the moral basis of confidentiality is protection of the client from harm (respect for client autonomy), the social function is the furtherance of the professional relationship – where there is no client trust there can be no professions.

Confidentiality can become corrupted into an overriding emphasis on protecting the power of the professional. This may lead to a justification for government interference in professional self-regulation, even substituting it with state regulation through the courts. Certainly self-regulation has its dangers and can degenerate into protectionism, but the other side of the coin is that self-regulation may be seen as a form of resistance against authoritarian centralisation.

Professor Stacey argues in Chapter 3 that professional privilege works against medical accountability. Self-regulation does not always work. In medicine 'clinical autonomy' means that each doctor is solely responsible for their patient, and if questioned then peer review is the only means available. The General Medical Council (GMC) does not appear to work satisfactorily at present, and clinical audit is not currently linked with discipline. Doctors are unique in possessing the privilege before law of having a determining voice – the so-called 'Bolam test'. There is also a privilege of clinical autonomy in hearing complaints, and even the Ombudsman cannot investigate the clinical aspects of a patient complaint. Stacey makes it clear that much needs to be changed. Disciplinary procedures, which might be invoked against doctors in defence of patients, are 'slow and cumbersome' and sometimes used 'against doctors who stand out against the system' as in the cases of Dr Wendy Savage and Dr Helen Zeitlin (p. 40).

Nursing also regulates itself, and somewhat more openly than medicine. The UKCC has shown a lot more concern about the health care professional's duty to disclose than the GMC has. For example, 'A Guide for Students of Nursing and Midwifery' (UKCC, 1992a) reminds students of their duty to bring 'patients' and clients' comments, both positive and negative, on the nature of the care received' to the person supervising their clinical experience or their teacher and ensure that the local procedures for handling complaints is observed. After all, student nurses, not yet socialised into the closed and hierarchical health care system, are often the first to blow the whistle. The most notable case of this occurred in 1992 when a large group of student nurses at St Bartholomew's College of Nursing expressed their anxieties about standards of care on the elderly wards to which they had been allocated for experience. Their letters of concern were not appreciated by management. Reg Pyne, the UKCC's officer for standards and ethics, was reported as saying that, 'I would be willing to excuse them for sending a letter that was not worded as delicately as some people would like if it had come from a group of young people who were extremely disturbed by what they had seen. They need guidance instead of criticism on such matters' (Eby, 1993).

The UKCC has also circulated an official letter on standards and the purchaser/provider contracts for hospitals and community health care services (UKCC, 1992b). It is stated here that purchasers should require that the nurses' Code of Professional Conduct be included in contracts of employment as a clause requiring compliance and that providers be able to demonstrate to the satisfaction of the purchaser their commitment to the Code. The letter also says that 'providers should recognise and honour the individual practitioner's right to freedom of speech consistent with the guidance issued by Government Health Departments'. (This guidance is examined in detail by Jean McHale in Chapter 10.) Indeed the UKCC publicly criticised the draft of this guidance, speaking of its 'threatening tone' and of its being 'heavily worded'.

In Chapter 4 Professor Orr emphasises how nursing now holds out the promise of becoming a more autonomous, professional and accountable discipline. Nurses are increasingly desirous of judging, making decisions and acting, questioning and challenging, without medical or managerial interference, but they face a daily struggle in institutions which appear very often to be moving in the opposite direction (see Hunt and Wainwright, 1994; Hunt, 1994, ch. 7).

Commercialisation will tend gradually to undermine the very notion of professional ethics as presently understood in medicine, nursing and the other health care professions. The nurses' regulatory body, the United Kingdom Central Council for Nursing, Midwifery and Health Visiting (UKCC), may publish advice about, for example, commercial sponsorship and advertising but how long will it be before such advice is ignored or treated with lip-service? (UKCC, 1990).

The crisis in health care provides a new opportunity for a debate about professionalism, and a new understanding of what a professional is or should be. If this opportunity is not seized then the professional will also be swallowed up by the market and will lose the traditional sense of social conscience and public service, which is surely worth saving, and take on the garb of the businessman or businessman's employee – and ironically do so at the very time when there is a felt need for reappraisal of our understanding of business management and corporate responsibility.

Politicians, managers, health carers

While in the traditional NHS managers were often, or usually, professional health carers who saw self-regulation as the principal disciplinary authority over their activities, things have now changed. Modern, non-clinical managers may not have much awareness of, or regard for, professional self-regulation. The new-style manager draws up an employment contract against a commercial background, and expects the health care professional to abide by it, even if that contract is at certain points apparently at variance with the health carer's professional rights and duties.

What is the manager to make of the professional understanding of confidentiality on the one hand, and the protection of the interests of the Trust or of the health authority on the other? Can management and clinical professionals work together with a similar understanding of confidentiality in the public interest? Is management, and indeed the legal system, prepared to move away from a presupposition in favour of confidentiality (or secrecy) to one in favour of a duty to disclose? Such a move would shift the burden from providing a 'public interest defence' for disclosure to providing a public interest ground for non-disclosure. Surely, this is what democracy requires.

As Ray Rowden suggests in Chapter 2, it is time that managers were made accountable, and subject to a professional code. Food for thought is provided by two sections of a recent and innovative code for managers:

> 4e. In the public interest, cooperate with others to uphold the law and to arrive at the truth in investigations and in disciplinary processes.
> 5c. Communicate to the public truthfully and without intent to mislead by slanting or suppressing information.
> (Institute of Management, 1992)

What we are witnessing is a power struggle between two strata: managers working with a commercial/industrial model and professionals working with a state welfare model. This reflects a wider power struggle in modern society between economic managers and welfare professionals (Perkins, 1989). A highly experienced and well-qualified health care professional and whistleblower told the researchers in Chapter 1: 'Clinicians are aware of a need, know what they want; the lay managers have a budget but cannot service the need, so tricks and devices are used to balance the two'.

It is unlikely that health care professionals, particularly doctors, will regain the power which was traditionally theirs. This does not mean that they must become subordinate to economic and financial managers ignorant of health care values and purposes. A new kind of health care professional, who is prepared to work across and even against traditional professional boundaries and rivalries, may yet be able to work with a new kind of publicly accountable manager. This will be possible only if management and administration in turn free themselves from political subordination so that all three – health care professionals, managers and politicians – are subject to democratic controls, including a separation of powers.

References

DoH (1992) *Report of the Committee of Inquiry into Complaints about Ashworth Hospital.* HMSO, London.

DOUGLAS, M. (1994) The Enforceability of 'Gagging' Clauses and Contracts. Unpublished paper, European Centre for Professional Ethics, University of East London and Brachers Solicitors.

EBY, M. (1993) The UKCC and the voicing of concerns. *The Whistle* 2, 8–9, Freedom to Care, West Molesey.

THE GUARDIAN (1990) Yours sincerely, F. G. Pink. *Society* supplement, 11th April, p. 21.

THE GUARDIAN (1992a) Waiting for Zeitlin. 14th August.

THE GUARDIAN (1992b) Bottomley Rejects Nurses' Plea to Ban Gagging Clauses. 28th April.

THE GUARDIAN (1994) The Bugging of an NHS Doctor (supplement). 1st April.

HUNT, G. (ed.) (1994) *Ethical Issues in Nursing.* Routledge, London.

HUNT, G. AND WAINWRIGHT, P. (eds) (1994) *Expanding the Role of the Nurse.* Blackwell Scientific, Oxford.

THE INDEPENDENT ON SUNDAY (1991) NHS Staff Gagged on Health Reforms. 12th May.

INSTITUTE OF MANAGEMENT (1992) *Code of Conduct and Guides to Professional Management Practice.* Institute of Management, London.

LABORATORY PRACTICE (1992) Fraud at Leeds. **41**(11), 8–10; Fraud at Leeds – 2. **41**(12), 36–7.

LENNANE, K. J. (1993) 'Whistleblowing': A Health Issue. *British Medical Journal* **307**, 11th September, 667–70.

MSF (1993) *News Release,* 22nd February, Manufacturing Science Finance, London.

NHS EXECUTIVE LETTER (1994) Dated 8th June 1994 from Personnel Directorate to Freedom to Care.

NHSME (1993) *Guidance for Staff on Relations with the Public and the Media.* NHSME, Leeds.

PERKINS, H. (1989) *The Rise of Professional Society*. Routledge, London.

UKCC (1989) *Exercising Accountability*. Advisory document, UKCC, London.

UKCC (1990) Statement on Advertising and Commercial Sponsorship. Issued with Registrar's letter 3/1990 dated 23rd April 1990, UKCC, London.

UKCC (1992a) A Guide for Students of Nursing and Midwifery. UKCC, London.

UKCC (1992b) Standards for Incorporation into Contracts for Hospital and Community Health Care Services. Registrar's Letter 37 (14/12/92), UKCC, London.

THE WHISTLE (1993) No. 2 (May), Freedom of Care, West Molesey.

THE WHISTLE (1993) No. 3 (November), Freedom to Care, West Molesey.

THE WHISTLE (1994) No. 4 (April), Freedom to Care, West Molesey.

Part One
The Actors

Part One

The A...

1

The whistleblowers speak

Geoffrey Hunt and Barbara Shailer

I am disappointed that one should find oneself having to prove one's competence and innocence simply because one upholds professional standards.
(Dismissed whistleblower's remark)

I would do it again. You cannot be a different person – you must stand by your moral and ethical code.
(Vindicated whistleblower's remark)

Introduction

A pilot survey of 30 whistleblowing health care professionals in the National Health Service in England was carried out by the European Centre for Professional Ethics, University of East London, in 1993. The object of the survey was to achieve some understanding of whistleblowers' concerns, the manner in which they attempt to address those concerns and the nature of the difficulties they encounter as a result.

We were interested in finding out whether there was a pattern, a story which goes beyond the unique experience of each. We think the answer is 'yes'. Beyond the biographical there are the outlines of a general narrative. At the individual level there is always the excuse, the claim that it is a one-off, a unique experience. When one begins to put all these individual cases together an account emerges which is about the kind of institutions in which individuals work or try to work.

The subjects were asked to fill in a questionnaire and they were interviewed face to face or, in some cases, over the telephone. The survey is not based on a random sample but on a convenience sample. The subjects had come to the researchers' attention through the media or through personal and professional contacts. To qualify for selection the subjects had to meet the following broad criteria: a member of the health care professions in the National Health Service in England who had, in their own perceptions, raised at least one concern about some important issue of policy, practice or standards and had as a result found themselves victimised or facing some form of hostility or obstruction. This is what is meant by the term 'whistleblower' in this study. (If, however, 'whistleblower' means someone who *goes public* then not all our respondents were whistleblowers. Some might consider 'obstructed complainant' to be a more accurate term for our respondents.)

Nearly all the subjects were nervous about the research and had to be given assurances of absolute confidentiality. Every effort has been made to remove from the data any identifying details. The 'Examples of Remarks' in this report should not be ascribed to any individual and are given here only to represent the *kind* of thing being said. For the sake of brevity there is some editing of the remarks.

Basic information

At the time at which the concern was expressed, five of the respondents were medical practitioners, 19 were nurses, three were midwives or health visitors and three were other professionals working in the National Health Service (NHS). Half were male and half female, 18 being in the 41–50 year old age group, eight in the 31–40 age group and four over 51 years of age. Thus the 'typical' whistleblower was about 40 years of age, a mature, well-qualified and experienced person at the height of his or her profession.

The respondents worked in 11 different health authorities at regional or equivalent level in England. Twenty three of the respondents were working in health authority managed units, but nearly all of these were at the time preparing for trust status. Four were working in trusts at the time they expressed their concerns. The other three were in units involving other bodies as well as the NHS. The method adopted ruled out the possibility of inferences about whether whistleblowing was more common in some regions than others.

The concerns were initiated over a 13 year period, some of them continuing to exercise those involved for five years or more. The breakdown for the years in which the complaint was initiated is as follows: 1980–84, five; 1985, one; 1986, one; 1987, two; 1988, four; 1989, one; 1990, six; 1991, seven; 1992, three. Although the numbers in this survey are too small to draw definite conclusions, one may put forward the hypothesis that a rash of whistleblowing broke out from 1990 suggesting a possible connection with the market reforms. Naturally, this issue is tied up with political perceptions.

Concerns and action taken

The respondents were asked what they had expressed concern about. This was posed as an open question and no suggestions were made to the subjects about kinds of concern. The categories below were compiled by the researchers from the data presented. (The same applies to the other categories listed in this report.) Some respondents had expressed concern about more than one matter.

Categories

Patient abuse	6
Inadequate care	12
Unethical research	3
Fraud/theft	4
Staff/resource shortage	10
Unfair treatment of staff member	3
Poor practice	4

Some had difficulty in identifying one factor because, we were made to understand, a situation of conflict often arises by degrees in a substandard or poorly managed environment. Sometimes an incident triggers off a major complaint and countercomplaints where tension has already been mounting for a considerable period. Thus in one case the 'trouble' seems to have started over the resuscitation equipment being too far away to be readily available in an emergency and in another a patient's lip bled when a colleague forced in a tablet.

We were interested in finding out what actions respondents had taken to get their concerns addressed, and what success they achieved. Obviously, the nature of the sample produces the results one would expect, to a large extent. If concerns had been addressed then they would not have been in our survey. Still, we are not interested in the fact that the concern was not addressed but in the manner in which it was not addressed. We want to learn something about *how* conflict arose, rather than *that* it arose (which we know already).

Respondents were asked what action they *first* took to get their concern addressed. Twenty six said that this had no effect and four that it had some effect.

Categories

Spoke/wrote to manager	19
Spoke to colleagues	5

Raised at meeting	4
Letter to personnel	1
Letter to health authority	1

Respondents were also asked what subsequent actions they took and whether these resulted in the concern being addressed. Subsequent actions were diverse. Most typically the employees continued up the management line, while others went next to a professional body or union for advice, often at the same time as following up management. Feeling obstructed at each level, some pursued the management line up to regional level, to the chair of the regional health authority and even on to the Secretary of State for Health. In some of the cases we examined, the persistence of the complainant resulted in police inquiries and prosecutions and in public inquiries which drew a great deal of media attention.

Again as one might expect, once the first expression of concern to a manager fails the employee who is persistent will tend to do several different things at more or less the same time and the issues become convoluted. The respondent finds themselves having to provide a defence against counterallegations while opening up new channels to make the original complaint and often having to make new complaints about the failures to respond to the original complaint. All kinds of parties might become involved: personnel officers, community health councils, specialist consumer groups, professional associations, regional medical officers, members of parliament, the police.

Naturally the complainant does not always pursue the original complaint in what, with hindsight, might be regarded as the most appropriate order or manner. Thus bringing in a union representative at quite an early stage tended in some cases to put higher management on the defensive and skipping a management level in lodging a complaint often caused ill feeling at that level. Respondents nearly always have an understandable account of why they did things in the order they did – very few were prepared to say 'Oh, that was a mistake, I should have done this before that'. The account generally depends on a grasp of the role based power relations involved in that situation, as well as the personal character of the principals. Thus a respondent might say something like, 'Although the procedure says I should have reported to x, if I had done that I would have been victimised, so I reported to y'.

It is significant, perhaps, how few of the respondents were able to point to any kind of collective action among the actions they took. Nearly everyone had at least one supportive colleague, but even this generally did not go beyond what one might call moral support. This outcome might be thought to have a lot to do with the nature of the sample – it was the 'lone wolf' that we interviewed. But we suspect that this explanation is too facile. Nearly everyone referred to fear, vulnerability and a conviction that nothing would change in any case. However, there were notable exceptions and two of our respondents in particular succeeded in rallying a large number of colleagues across different disciplines.

The quantity and nature of the evidence obtained by the employee to support the case being made was very variable. In some cases, believing that management (usually at a low level) would readily believe what the complainant had to say the complainant made little effort to gather evidence in any form. Faced with unexpected rebuttals the complainant then found themselves at a disadvantage in making the case. Going back to gather evidence, they then found that it had been 'concealed'.

On the other hand, some had as much evidence as anyone could reasonably require including, in some cases, official and independent audits. This did not necessarily make things easier. Evidence from an audit report was, in one case, concealed and an employee told in no uncertain terms not to reveal it. In other cases evidence was 'explained away' or simply ignored.

Many of the respondents felt that by taking their complaint further they only succeeded in getting their concern aired internally – as though discussion were some kind of psychological therapy for the employee rather than a means of establishing the truth of the matter and solutions to problems identified. Other management responses varied from a plea for 'help' in 'avoiding trouble' to 'screaming and shouting'.

Several respondents were disappointed with their unions, because the more difficult things got the more they tended to side with management, in the eyes of the complainant. In other words, respondents, with a few exceptions, felt that the unions did not really help them to get the concern addressed. This claim seems to us to be perfectly justified in the cases we examined. At the same time many reported to us that they only felt they were getting somewhere with their concern when they involved an external or quasi-external body such as a community health council or a consumer group.

Availability and effectiveness of procedures

In a separate section of the questionnaire employees were asked more formally about the procedures or pathways they followed. Respondents were asked about 14 procedures which they might have used in expressing their concerns. These questions were closed (i.e. choices were presented beforehand). Questions were asked about the availability of these procedures and about their effectiveness on a scale of completely effective, largely effective, slightly effective, completely ineffective.

Respondents were asked whether they took their concerns to: a workplace meeting (e.g. at ward level), the grievance procedure, management, the personnel officer, an ombudsman, a union, a professional body, the disciplinary procedure, the health authority, the health and safety officer, a statutory regulatory body, the media, a Member of Parliament, a consumers' group or some other body.

The ranking of the procedures (in descending order of number using it) is as follows:

1. manager;
2. workplace meeting;
3. union;
4. health authority;
5. MP;
6. media;
7. professional body, grievance procedure;
8. regulatory body;
9. personnel officer, consumers' group;
10. disciplinary procedure, ombudsman;
11. other;
12. safety officer.

The vast majority (23) took their concern to a workplace meeting such as a ward or multidisciplinary meeting at some stage or other and of these 18 found it completely ineffective or only slightly effective in addressing their concern while the other five found it completely or largely effective.

About one third (11) used the local grievance procedure and a slightly larger number (13) did not use it even though they knew it was available. No one thought it had any real effectiveness, for all of them considered it completely ineffective in dealing with their concern or only slightly so.

All the complainants contacted management at some stage, either verbally or in writing, some submitting official reports. An overwhelming majority regarded this as completely ineffective or only of slight effect in getting the matter addressed (that is, 23 said it was ineffective and six slightly effective). In fact, only one was quite satisfied with the manager's response, although even that one decided to take the matter further.

Nine respondents contacted the personnel officer at some point and the same proportion did not do so although they knew this was available to them. The remainder did not think of it or did not consider it relevant. A large majority (eight) of those who used this procedure thought it was completely ineffective or only slightly effective.

Regarding an ombudsman (such as the health commissioner), most people did not think of this or did not consider it relevant. However, eight did contact the appropriate ombudsman at some stage and of these six found it completely ineffective or only of slight effect while two found this to have some useful effect.

Only two respondents did not belong to a union. Six different unions were involved at the time. (There have been mergers since.) Eighteen contacted a union and nine did not do so even though they knew one was available to them. A number of respondents belonged at some point to two unions, turning away from one they found ineffective to one which they then found effective. Of those who used a union, about twice as many found it ineffective or only slightly effective as found it completely or largely effective.

Thirteen of the respondents consulted their professional body (which in some cases was a branch of their union). Ten found this to be completely ineffective or of slight effect while three found it completely or largely effective.

Eight of the respondents attempted to use a local disciplinary procedure against a colleague or manager at some stage, but seven found it completely ineffective and the other only slightly effective.

Seventeen of the respondents wrote to their health authority at district or regional level to inform them of their concern and/or complain about the local response to their expression of concern. Only three respondents found this to be completely or largely effective, 12 finding it to be ineffective and two of slight effectiveness.

Regarding the health and safety officer, this was not thought of or was not regarded as relevant by quite a few respondents. About half knew it was available but did not use it. Four respondents did report matters to this officer, two of them finding it completely or largely effective and the other two ineffective or of slight effect.

The General Medical Council (GMC) and the United Kingdom Central Council for Nursing, Midwifery and Health Visiting (UKCC) were the appropriate statutory regulatory bodies for all but three of the respondents. Ten of the respondents contacted one of these two in the course of pursuing their complaint. Five considered the body ineffective and two slightly effective in dealing with the matter, while the other three considered it completely or largely effective.

Thirteen of the respondents contacted the local or national media at some point in pursuing their concern. Every one of these had first used some channel internal to their organisation to lodge their complaint. Twelve of those who used the media considered this to be completely or largely effective in getting their concern addressed.

Exactly half of the respondents had gone to their MP about the matter at some stage. Six considered it completely ineffective and five slightly so, while three considered it to have been completely effective and one largely effective in getting the concern addressed.

The category of 'consumer groups' included consumer health councils and various patient/client 'watchdogs'. Nearly a third (nine) approached such a group with their concern at some stage or other and they were about equally divided as to the effectiveness of having done so.

Examples of other actions taken to get a concern addressed were: informing a funding body, consulting a professional grouping (e.g. professors), using patients' complaints procedure. Six of the respondents took some action which does not fall among the 14 procedures listed above. Four of these found this action to be completely effective.

Obstacles

Respondents were asked: Did you encounter any obstacles (from management) in expressing concern and if so what were they? In the course of expressing concern, was a complaint made against you and if so what? The answers give a rough picture of what the respondents took to be the *resistance* to getting their concerns addressed. Again, the fact that all say they encountered obstacles is not surprising, since if they had encountered no obstacles they would, presumably, not be part of this study. What is interesting is the *nature* of the obstacles.

About one third reported various forms of intimidation, including warnings about career prospects and continuing employment; one third reported that the major obstacle was simply passivity or disbelief, with their concerns being ignored. Three said their suspension prevented them pursuing their concern. Three said they received threats of violence from colleagues implicated in allegations; four said that they were put under surveillance by management; three that they were labelled as sick or 'unable to cope'; two complained of management and senior colleagues 'closing ranks' against them; one reported being moved out of their office on a pretext; another reported that a warning was made that 'someone else would do the work' if they 'didn't want to'; two complained at cover-up measures; one that the caseload kept changing unreasonably as a consequence of the complaint.

Seven of the respondents said that no official countercomplaint had been made against them but most of the others had ended up before a disciplinary hearing at some level. The most common countercomplaint was 'unprofessional conduct' and this broke down into vague accusations ranging from 'being uncooperative' or 'making trouble' to the more specific such as (most commonly) 'not complying with management's instructions' and 'breaching confidentiality'. Two said that their principal offence, it was claimed, was having 'damaged the reputation' of their institution. Three were accused of abusing or neglecting patients, after they had themselves lodged complaints about colleagues abusing or neglecting patients. The sexual conduct or preferences of the complainants were questioned by colleagues and management in three cases, while in several cases the sources of 'the problem' was said by management to be that the complainant was too sick or weak to 'cope' and they were treated as medically unfit.

Managers receptive?

Respondents were asked in an open question if management was on the whole receptive to the expression of concerns. The categories are drawn from the data presented. Four reported that the managers they approached might have helped but were constrained by *their* superiors.

Categories

Constrained by higher level managers	4
Ignored, sent complainant to Coventry	4
Made threats, victimised	7
Failed to answer letters	2
Denial, defensiveness, lies	6
Buck-passing	2

Examples of remarks

'Immediate managers were supportive, but undermined from above.'
'They did not answer letters, told me not to write any more.'
'They attempted to explain things away; ambivalence and excuses.'
'Did not listen, told lies.'
'Immediate managers receptive, but seniors showed hostility, denial and anger at meetings.'
'Initial interest, but nothing was investigated.'
'Local managers were threatened with dismissal if they supported me.'
'They pretended to hold discussions but resolved nothing.'

Union support

Respondents were asked in an open question whether they had consulted a union and whether it had been helpful.

Categories

Turned against complainant	2
One unhelpful, next helpful	5
Very helpful	5
Totally unhelpful	7
Limited help, no follow-through	6

Examples of remarks

'Pretended to help, pressured us, then let us down.'
'Very supportive.'
'One was useless, but the other very helpful.'
'Supportive, but no legal representation offered.'
'Limited help, stopped managerial intimidation, but no follow-up, and
   after my dismissal the union wasn't effective.'
'Extremely well represented by my union.'

Support of colleagues

Respondents were asked in an open question if they were supported by
their colleagues and whether colleagues were hostile. Some reported
that junior colleagues or peers were supportive while senior ones were
unsupportive.

Categories

Majority supportive	10
Majority unsupportive	17
Junior yes/senior no	3
Hostility in some form	19
Fear mentioned	6

Examples of remarks

'Colleagues felt threatened and exposed.'
'The majority privately supportive, but departmentally unsupportive,
   they felt intimidated, although only one was hostile.'
'Many signed a petition, but frightened of further action.'
'They became collegiate when chips were down.'

'They were frightened for their jobs and pensions.'
'A reluctance to communicate.'

Going public

The questionnaire contained this question: Did you (at any stage) take your concern outside your organisation? If so, to whom and why?

Seventeen said they did take their concern outside and 13 said they did not do so at any stage. Of those who did, 15 took the initiative themselves and felt that they had no alternative. They felt that they had made every effort to get the issue addressed internally and had been obstructed and that therefore they were justified in going outside the organisation in getting a matter of serious public concern addressed. In the other two cases it was the press who first approached the complainant, having learned about the matter from another source. Having been approached, the complainants did not feel it was wrong to confirm publicly the concern they had expressed internally. 'Going outside' does not necessarily mean first going to the media. As we noted earlier, 13 did at some point speak to the media, but for most of these this was a last resort. Some of them had already been to bodies which were, so to speak, one foot outside their own organisation such as a district medical or nursing officer or the appropriate community health council and others had already spoken in confidence to their MP. Employee perceptions as to what counted as 'going outside' were quite often different from employer perceptions. Thus some managers thought that informing the recognised union was 'going outside' while the employee thought this was still 'inside'. The same goes for contacting a regulatory body such as the UKCC. More surprisingly, perhaps, some employers seem to have thought (according to the respondent concerned) that it was 'going outside' (and therefore wrong) to contact the police, even in cases where there was *prima facie* evidence of criminal wrongdoing (fraud, theft, physical abuse of patients).

Some did not contact the press simply because it was inappropriate. Those who did not contact the press did not, for the most part, think it would have been wrong to do so. Instead they did not do so either because they did not trust the press to get the story right or because they felt it would jeopardise their jobs.

Examples of remarks

Some remarks made in justification of going outside were:
'Because of the internal obstacles.'
'Due to nil action from district or regional health authority.'

'Because I was fobbed off and then victimised.'
'Over six months of raising the concern internally had failed.'
'Nobody was listening to me.'
'It became clear to me that the health authority would do nothing unless pressured (and probably not even then).'

Personal consequences

Respondents were asked an open question about the long term consequences for them as individuals of having expressed concern over standards of care.

Categories

Lost job/resigned	16
Promotion blocked	4
Financial difficulties	11
Marital/relationship/family difficulties	11
Made sick	4
Made career change	5
Enhanced respect/self-esteem	4
Reinstated	3
Re-employment difficulties	3
Depression/anxiety	4

Examples of remarks

'A great stress to my family.'
'My career is in limbo.'
'I was offered a non-job, I felt burnt out.'
'The experience hardened my inner resolve.'
'It was very upsetting, it made me ill.'
'I was labelled as the person who'll "grass on colleagues".'
'I can't find work because I'm now seen as a potential troublemaker.'

Consequences for workplace

Respondents were asked an open question about the long term consequences for their workplace. The respondents appeared to be about equally divided as to whether their whistleblowing had led to improvements or not. Most of those who thought there were improvements thought that they were minor or cosmetic. Respondents were about equally divided as to whether their perceived 'opponents' (the people complained against or the managers they felt had obstructed their expression of concern) had been adversely affected by the whistleblowing, i.e. whether they had been disciplined or moved, for example. Five felt the experience had made their colleagues more questioning and assertive, while 10 reported a subsequent climate of fear, low morale and attempts to gag.

There were notable failures and equally notable successes. In the worst cases the complainant had lost their job or resigned in disgust with little or no attention having been given to the concern raised. In some cases there had been obvious if small improvements, while in others the improvements were more subtle, improvements being made without any acknowledgement that these had resulted from the whistleblowing. It was felt by some that unacknowledged improvements were a way of containing the situation without appearing to be 'weak' and giving encouragement to more 'troublemakers'. There was no acknowledgement that it would in general be a good idea to listen to staff. In other cases the whistleblower had retained or regained their job and succeeded in achieving a large part of their aims and in one case the success was total. (We cannot go into detail without identifying people.)

In half a dozen cases the employee took the employer to an industrial tribunal and at the eleventh hour the employer would offer larger and larger sums of money to settle the matter out of court until the employee (by now exhausted and financially ruined) accepted. Although the employer would say that this was to avoid further unnecessary expense, it was felt by the employee that management was afraid to be proved wrong in public. This would have repercussions relating to extension of media attention, and also open an avenue for the reception of other concerns over falling standards.

Examples of remarks

'Low morale, distrust of management, the abuse continues.'
'Colleagues now annoyed and frightened.'
'Some gains but did not get more staff.'
'Gagging clauses added to job descriptions, intimidation and fear still evident, opponents moved but new managers have same approach.'
'Staff intimidated, frightened to complain.'
'Some colleagues have been enabled to make a stand, but the impact on the institution was small.'
'Concerns over standards have run underground, staff are frightened for their jobs.'
'Management has taken steps to avoid leaks of what is happening.'
'It was painful, but we got management to listen in the end.'

Disappointed?

Respondents were asked whether they were on the whole disappointed by their experience and if so, by what in particular. Some expressed 'moral shock' in the sense of surprise and anguish at the dishonesty, lack of integrity, cowardice, etc. of some of those involved.

Categories

Disappointed at colleagues	10
Disappointed at management	10
A positive learning experience	3
Moral shock	11

Examples of remarks

'Disappointed by lack of action and their disbelief in me.'
'I was made a scapegoat by management, this should not happen in 1993.'
'Feeling of hopelessness over standards of care, with silenced work-force.'
'Feel very bitter about treatment by managers after all that hard work and effort.'
'Saddened by compliance and inertia of colleagues.'
'Disappointed that injustices remain and bad working practices continue.'
'Disappointed that managers can be so unprincipled.'
'Disappointed that power is unbridled in public bodies.'

Easier?

Respondents were asked this question: In retrospect, if one thing could have made things easier what would it have been?

Categories

Listening, investigative, pro-active management	9
Support from union	1
Support from colleagues	4

Independent body/forum	10
Proper procedure for expressing concerns	10
An open ethos	3
Support from regulatory body	1
Respect for competence/clinical priority	5

Examples of remarks

'If management had been prepared to investigate and act in the first instance.'
'Professionals need better representation on health authorities.'
'Proper procedures and forum for addressing issues of care.'
'A democratic and consultative ethos, with policies clearly defined for *patient care*, with an acknowledgement of the experience and values of all professionals involved.'
'If colleagues had been united in presenting case to management.'
'Legislation to protect from retribution those expressing concern.'
'An independent and impartial body to appeal to.'
'Openness and a focus on the clinical priorities.'

Do it again?

Respondents were asked if they would raise concerns over matters of this nature again and if they would, whether they would do it differently. Twenty seven said they would raise such concerns again, one said no and two were not sure.

The one who said no added, 'It cost me my health, my family's health and happiness, and I would be concerned about the effects on other members of staff'. The remarks made in support of the positive replies are very interesting:

Examples of remarks

'It is a personal commitment to maintain decency in care.'
'However, I would need to know I was protected by some outside organisation.'
'There has to be a sense of justice for nurses and patients.'
'It would let down the profession if no action were taken.'
'There must be humane treatment of patients.'
'I am here to serve the public; I owe it to them to give my knowledge and concern.'

'I cannot witness distress and not speak out.'

'Hospitals should not be hazardous to health.'

'Nothing is gained by keeping quiet – no problem is solved that way.'

'The truth must be told, patients must be protected and bad managers exposed and the professional code upheld.'

'Progress must be made; we appear to be going backwards.'

'I could not live with it otherwise; I cannot tolerate glossing over problems to protect the institution's interests.'

'I would like to be able to, because honesty and integrity requires it, but I would consider the options very carefully as the process can be very destructive.'

On the question of whether they would do it differently next time exactly half said they would not do it differently, 14 said they would and one expressed uncertainty. This is surprising, perhaps, because one might expect a majority to have 'learned from their mistakes'. In fact, the majority believed that in the circumstances there was very little of significance which they could have done differently in getting their concern addressed with a minimum of fuss. And of those who would do things differently, most thought they should have been more rather than less assertive. We have the impression that most (but not all) of the complainants now believe that if they were going to raise a concern of a serious nature in a similar institution then an ascending spiral of obstruction and victimisation is all they could expect. The only alternative was not to raise the concern at all.

The most common remark in this connection, made by seven respondents, was that a formal complaint would be lodged much *earlier* if they found themselves in a similar situation again. It seems that quite a few thought that they had become bogged down in difficulties because they had left things too late and had not been well prepared with their case. They had believed that the evidence was obvious enough and that their views would be respected and were surprised and frustrated when that did not happen.

Examples of remarks

'There was no other way to gain the outcome wanted.'

'I might have approached things in a more subtle way.'

'I would have tried to predict all the ways management would respond, so that I would have been 100% prepared with a good case for them.'

'I would have left and not complained.'

'I tried to be understanding, but I should have screamed from the first.'

'I should have gone to the press earlier.'
'I would be more cautious and not make myself so vulnerable.'

Methodological limitations

The methodological limitations of this survey are obvious enough. It was intended as a pilot, that is, as an exploratory preamble to more extensive and rigorous research.

The sample was small and was not randomly selected. The study lacks any control by which comparisons can be made. There is no reference to:

a) a group which did not express concerns although it had some which might have been expressed;
b) a group which did not have any concerns to express;
c) a group which expressed concerns and had them properly addressed, in their own perceptions.

In the absence of such comparisons one cannot be very definite about what characterizes a 'whistleblowing' situation.

One reviewer of this study asked us whether it shows, or can show, whether the problem lies in how the expressed concerns were received rather than in the character of the complainants. Our reply to this is that whatever the character of the complainant, in any accountable institution one would expect proper procedures and a willingness to investigate concerns raised. Although it is quite possible that some of the respondents may have been 'difficult' people, this does not satisfactorily explain the *institutional* difficulties they encountered in trying to raise concerns which were of a serious character. It would be much too bizarre to try to explain away every obstacle as a deficiency in the character of the whistleblower if not least because many of them were completely or partly vindicated in public.

It is clear that no conclusions can be drawn from this survey about the general incidence of whistleblowing in the UK National Health Service. It is impossible on the basis of this study alone to know how far any of our findings are generalisable. Of course, there is a great deal of relevant background evidence (to which we do not refer) in terms of related studies, anecdotes and personal experiences, newspaper and journal reports, claims made by unions, professional bodies, consumer groups and politicians to suggest that much of what we have found is not unusual in today's health service.

Then there is the question of perceptions. Connected with this is the retrospective character of the accounts given by the respondents. Interpretations of events will be contested and both whistleblowers and the various authorities involved may 'rationalise', consciously or unconsciously, to justify their acts and omissions. In this study one hears one side of the story. Still, this is perhaps the side that is not heard so often and so clearly.

Conclusion

Despite the methodological limitations we think an outline narrative emerges which is worth considering, suggesting stimulating lines of inquiry and discussion.

Against a background of low or damaged self-esteem among clinical staff (often nurses, but increasingly doctors too) in which the professional carer's view is not respected or even sought and working in a general climate of fear, a major incident which is professionally 'unbearable' leads to the dogged pursuit of a complaint by someone with a little more courage than most or less to lose than most. Typically, the whistleblower would be told by colleagues that they were 'right', but that it was futile or too risky to complain. Unions presented themselves as weak and unwilling to follow through. The complainant would find themselves out on a limb.

The professional would regard themselves as working in a situation which was morally unacceptable and this perception of unacceptability, originating in and reinforced by the standards of a professional code or tradition, would appear to be flouted, offending the professional's sense of integrity. The traditions are those of public service, rising above impartiality and gift or favour, and the autonomous setting, monitoring and defence of standards which have been cultivated through decades of professional experience.

The respondents were quite clear in identifying the object of the whistleblowing – health care research distorted or rendered useless by inducements, levels of staffing and facilities so low as to threaten or nullify customary standards of care, impending closure of units or beds, the abuse or neglect of patients by colleagues who fall below professional expectations, theft and fraud. In every case there was a preparedness to present evidence in some shape or form and in nearly all cases the matter raised ought not (we believe) to have been controversial – many respondents pointed to (some independent) audit reports, quality assurance exercises and incident reports to back up their claims.

Professionals with a serious concern would find themselves frustrated at every step in the internal procedures of accountability, countercomplaints would often be made against the complainant and the disagreement would escalate until the complainant felt there was no alternative but to go public. The complainant would now be at serious risk of losing their job.

In conclusion, our study suggests that some hostilities between management and the caring professions over matters of standards arise not because the concerns about standards are *unfounded*, but because of a reluctance on the part of those with managerial responsibilities to *establish* in a fair and cooperative spirit whether or not the concerns are unfounded.

2

Managerial accountability

Andrew Wall and Ray Rowden

Part One

Andrew Wall

Twenty years ago 'accountability' was subsumed u der other concepts such as responsibility and chain of command. In a standard management text we find the statement:

> ... accountability is really an aspect of responsibility ... the latter term has much wider currency in management practice.
>
> (Kootz and O'Donnell, 1972)

The assumption which underpinned public sector management at that time might have been sufficiently secure to deflect closer analysis. Today public scrutiny of what public servants do is far greater. Does this suggest a loss of confidence in the standards that public servants bring to their work or is it just that the public now have a greater interest in the management of those services funded directly out of the public purse?

Both views are sustainable. In the National Health Service there has been a steady decline in public confidence, as recorded in a yearly survey (Davies, 1991). Associated with this is the increasing confusion in the mind of the public regarding the organisational changes following the most recent reforms. The impression is that whatever the difficulties facing the NHS, they are compounded by a burgeoning and increasingly unaccountable bureaucracy. No phone-in radio programme on the topic of the NHS will escape criticisms of the supposed large number of managers. Attempts to justify the current position by explaining the increased transaction costs of the new system of contracting will scarcely placate these critics. There are also disturbing reports of large scale financial scandals which, even where they have not involved criminal activity, have nevertheless demonstrated gross mismanagement.

Inside the organisation matters do not appear to be any better. The changes brought about by the 1990 reforms have led to an unparalleled clear-out of senior staff and the mood of those remaining is one of personal anxiety; no longer is the NHS a safe place to be employed. Standards of employer/employee relationships have decayed in a manner which would have seemed inconceivable 20 years ago.

Something has clearly shaken the belief that those working in the NHS have an unambiguous view of what they are accountable for and to whom. However, it would be unfair merely to lay the responsibility for this state of affairs at the door of the managers themselves. Something about the climate in which they now work has had a profound effect on the way they behave. This chapter aims to explore the context of the NHS manager's work and to offer some hope for redeeming the situation so that managers have a clearer view of their duty to the public, a view understood by the community at large.

Public accountability

It has frequently been observed that there is considerable confusion regarding accountability in the public sector (Day and Klein, 1987; Starks, 1991; Massey, 1993). Are we talking about the line of command from Parliament through ministers and their ministries down into the field or are we more concerned with serving our clients and patients and the communities in which they live? Neither of these conceptions covers the relationship professionals have with their regulating bodies, which will be for them more compelling than relatively intangible ideas such as being answerable to the local community. In fact, all these 'masters' have to be served in one way or the other and the dilemma health service managers face is how best to do this, especially when there may be conflicting imperatives.

At the top

Simply stated, health service managers are accountable through the hierarchy to the Secretary of State for Health. They are there to implement the policies of the government of the day which has been elected to govern the country's affairs. But is to govern the same as to manage? It could be argued that recent governments have confused the two, leading to centralised decision making and incurring the frustration of managers and sometimes their contempt for politicians.

But the politicians are in a dilemma. Through the process of parliamentary questions and, even more demanding, through the Public Accounts Committee and the Select Committee for Health, very specific matters can be raised and brought before the public. Ministers anxious to protect their reputations will endeavour to ensure that the civil servants protect them against having no answer in such circumstances. It could be said that this process does not enhance public accountability but merely trivialises it. However, this is to dismiss it too easily, for many items discussed in the Select Committee would have been hidden for one reason or another within the organisation. Sometimes these reasons are creditable, but perhaps more often there is a simple desire not to cause embarrassment to the minister or to create a supposed loss of confidence in the public perception of the NHS.

If we accept the right of the minister to call for information of any kind, does that mean that the local managers have always to give that work priority? Not necessarily. It cannot be sensible to skew operational management in such a way. But the local manager must give full reasons why he or she is unable to comply. Proper behaviour therefore demands that the civil servants protecting their minister do not then use their authority in a threatening manner but equally that the local manager does not unreasonably withhold information which is accessible.

Such an interpretation may well be challenged by the Chief Executive to the NHS Management Executive (NHSME) on the grounds that, in the new NHS, the NHSME is the head of the organisation. The authority for this view is ambiguous. Technically, the Chief Executive is a permanent secretary within the civil service (but second in rank to the policy permanent secretary in the Department of Health). It could be argued, therefore, that the NHSME Chief Executive can *ask* but he cannot *tell* the managers in the field, whose employers are the various health authorities. At the next level down the situation is a little clearer in that regions have a duty to require district and Family Health Services authorities to be accountable by making reports on their work and the associated expenditure. But this does not make the region the legal employer of the DHA or FHSA staff. Unfortunately this has not stopped some regions from indulging in patronage, leaning heavily on DHAs and FHSAs in the matter of removing staff from employment under the guise of organisational change.

We may learn that accountability through the hierarchy is secured as much through informal but powerful influences as it is through invoking statutory relationships. This threatens the safeguarding of standards.

Health authorities

Another problem arises when a local health authority defines its main accountability as being to its local community. That members of an authority's board should hold this view is not surprising given the way the board's non-executive members are nominated. There is an emphasis in that process on the importance of bringing personal skills and local knowledge to the benefit of the NHS in a particular community. The absence of an electoral method of selecting non-executives to boards does not seem to decrease the sense of obligation those non-executives feel towards their community; rather the reverse. However, a difficulty arises when the local community has a different agenda from that of the government. The rhetoric of consultation has been set out by the government itself (DoH, 1992). But it would seem that in a tussle between local demands and central requirements, the centre is likely to win. This is so if only for the dubious reason that pressure is put on local managers to ensure compliance if they personally are not to suffer. For instance, a DHA which, after consultation with its local community, came out with a clear mandate to continue with the provision of community hospitals even though that restricted the amount of money available for reducing waiting lists was told not to 'play politics' by the Regional General Manager.

It will be said, no doubt, that this sort of case is seldom as clearcut and that the DHA was 'motivated' to challenge the authority of the region as well as to represent their community. True accountability could therefore be said to be demonstrated by not creating this sort of organisational infighting. But this in turn seems a little dishonest. The dilemma was a real one and calls fundamentally into question whether the Secretary of State is master or servant. Ultimately, the government is there to do what the electorate want and if they will not or cannot then they must expect to be removed at the ballot box. Certainly, for practical purposes, in a country which is nervous of referenda, the government has to make many assumptions if it is to make any progress at all. Despite this, heavyhanded use of authority down the line is unlikely to increase general confidence that the public interest is being served and is in any case pernicious in the way it stifles innovation and good practice among public service managers.

Efficiency, effectiveness, responsiveness

Managers have on their part to demonstrate good practice. Efficiency, effectiveness and responsiveness are the criteria which are now commonly used to assess the overall performance of management. For health service managers to be able to demonstrate them requires considerable effort. Efficiency, for instance, is not just a question of speed of delivery. Speed is sometimes of the essence, say, in a recovery room, but at other times speed would positively impede the progress of a patient painstakingly treading the path towards recovery. The efficient use of resources is something which can be shown to the public by means of comparative statements and performance indicators, but these need some inside knowledge to interpret. Time wasted in the operating theatre waiting for a recalcitrant surgeon is not immediately obvious, but there is no reason why this should not be known through the publication of numbers of patients per list and similar comparators. Intermediaries may be needed such as the Community Health Council. If efficiency is difficult to assess, effectiveness is even more so. Crude comparisons such as mortality rates after surgery need very careful presentation if they are not to give the wrong impression. Nevertheless, they can be revealing, as is a great deal of outcome information. It is the work of the provider unit's board to expose the information to open discussion. Trust boards may feel nervous in doing so because adverse reports may ruin their market. In this and other respects the competitiveness in the market approach can prove an obstacle to accountability. The pro-marketeers would no doubt argue that inefficiency and ineffectiveness are punished in the market by failure and that is accountability enough. But as the failure of a part of the health service may be beyond what is politically tolerable, the discipline of the market is considerably compromised.

Lastly, health service managers have to demonstrate responsiveness. They have a duty to the patients to ensure not only that the service is effective and that the patients are dealt with in an orderly and timely fashion, but also that patients are treated with a respect for their individuality. For many users this will be the most telling test of the accountability of the NHS. Is the organisation still able to see him or her as a person with a unique set of needs? A great deal of effort is going into convincing patients that the NHS has improved in this respect and quality initiatives are now being universally applied. Building confidence takes time, however, and some of the interventions fail to be more than skindeep. True accountability to the public is secured by a reputation which can only be assured by meeting standards over a considerable period.

Assuring accountability

Contracts

On the face of it the new arrangements in the NHS should make accountability more transparent. As relationships between levels of the NHS are now based on contracts, purchasers of services now need only *specify* and providers will perform accordingly. But this simplification conceals considerable dangers and may, as some people believe to be already the case, lead to a less accountable service than before. At the most obvious level, if the specification is incomplete then certain things do not get done. In any case, is it reasonable to specify exactly how to behave in all circumstances? A recent case where an elderly patient was tied to a sanichair and left and subsequently died would not have been avoided by a more complete specification. And yet it is exactly this sort of incident which the public wish to be assured will not happen.

Another problem with the contractual relationship is that it tends to be concerned primarily with *what* gets done rather than *how*. Trusts have to date been resistant to interference from purchasers as to how they should manage their affairs. For instance, it has been considered inappropriate to make any observations over the style of staff management even though this is clearly related to the well-being of patients. One way out of this ends-dominated approach would be to develop more sensitive processes of accreditation or regulation. Purchasers, in their role as advocates of the communities they serve, should have a responsibility for seeing that the providers have standards which are acceptable and would not invite criticism from the public. Precontract review of providers can enhance the relationship between the purchasers by developing a sense of partnership and thereby reducing the conflict inherent in the contracting process. The public are not edified by public disagreement on the terms of a contract. They might be more reassured to know that even before the contract was being discussed, the purchaser had checked some of the crucial standards relating to patient care.

Managers have a particular responsibility to demonstrate compliance with statutory provisions. In this respect the NHS record is not particularly good. Adherence to the requirements of the Health and Safety at Work Act has sometimes been compromised by the overriding demands of patient care. It is hard to spend money on fire escapes rather than more surgical operations. However, when patients and staff lose their lives in a fire the public are quick to allocate blame. A developing awareness of risk management helps managers to show that they accept their obligations to observe the law.

Corporate governance

The proper performance of boards – corporate governance – is now a priority, given recent scandals. Boards have to demonstrate that they operate in the public interest as the custodians of public funds. The tendency of boards to conduct a considerable amount of business in private threatens public accountability.

Transparency has its problems too. The media, always anxious for newsworthy copy, can impede and waylay management and distort priorities.

Public affairs are no longer necessarily run by public bodies. This has come about because bureaucracies have a reputation for being inflexible and wasteful. For this reason the Conservative governments of the last few years have encouraged the fragmentation of welfare organisation in the belief that smaller and better focused businesses will be intrinsically more efficient. The setting up of agencies has occurred across the whole of the public sector, even including the civil service. Within the NHS the regions have been reduced in size so that many functions previously managed directly within the hierarchy now operate with considerable freedom outside it, in some cases becoming privatised. Does this development compromise public accountability?

The NHS has always used private contractors for some work, usually work such as window cleaning which can be easily specified. But the opting out of computer and information services has proved to be quite another matter. The clients, in the shape of RHAs and DHAs, have difficulty in drawing up specifications in a situation where innovation is required to find solutions to problems. So the contractor has two roles, one as management consultant and the other as supplier of goods. If the contractor is to be effective in the former role then a longer term relationship needs to be developed. This may lead in turn to some compromising of those standing orders which require all work to be submitted to a tendering procedure. It is a moot point whether rigid adherence to standing orders will prove cheaper than developing an ongoing relationship with a particular supplier. And how is the public to know, given that the managers themselves are in doubt?

The role of the board is crucial to the management of this situation. The board acts as the safeguard of the public interest by a thorough examination of the proposals and obtaining expert advice. It cannot be acceptable for chairpersons or chief executives to take unilateral action, as this impugns their reputations. Corporate decision making cannot absolutely protect the public against wrongdoing but it goes far in assuring the public that every effort has been made not to expose public interest to undue risk.

Personal accountability

Consumerism

Much has to be done to restore public confidence in the manner in which the NHS is run. Both an understanding of the political environment and a regard for proper procedures will do much, but there is still something missing. How can the public be sure that health service managers and the non-executives who work with them will know what is the right way to behave? The political context in which they now work has emphasised the consumerist model to such an extent that it would appear that keeping the customer happy is all that is required. The inadequacy of such a view must be obvious. Reducing the responsibility of a public service to the ability merely to react to consumer demand ultimately disempowers the people working in that service and provides no opportunity for leadership. We know that without vision, without a sense of direction, organisations decay. To condemn the NHS to a philosophy of consumerism is to serve the public badly. As has been said:

> People are citizens first, and mere consumers a poor second; if governments are to be held accountable, this relationship of the individual to the state must remain.

> (Massey, 1993)

Values

Values are paramount. But whose and how are they determined? Health service managers usually work with utilitarian assumptions and may describe their obligation as one of maximising benefits to the greatest number of patients. Doctors and other professionals may find this view at odds with their responsibility to their individual patient. For them the patient has the right to treatment and it is improper for a manager to interfere with that professional duty. Sticking rigidly to this position is not possible in a cash limited service and, indeed, to do so could result in other patients being denied care and treatment.

We may assume that all but a handful of people in the NHS feel a duty to patients – they have some sense of wanting to help others. Is this sense not enough to ensure their proper behaviour? It might be but for the weightiness and sharpness of some of the dilemmas they face. How will a sense of duty help sort priorities which may result in one patient getting nothing? Some people are tempted to make choices by assessing the worthiness of the patient but this is fraught with dangers, leading to discriminatory judgements being made about lifestyle or social usefulness.

Given these problems, how are managers to respond to the need to be accountable to the public for their decisions? At a crude level, asking the public to choose between a baby and an elderly person is to invite sentimental responses in favour of one or the other from which there can be no guarantee of a sensible answer. But if the public are not to be involved, how are these life and death decisions to be made?

In the NHS, and maybe in health systems everywhere, this discussion is only just beginning. Accountability requires that managers set out the choices to be made, indicate who is to be involved in their evaluation and how the decisions are finally to be made. Public confidence is sometimes undermined by a lack of clarity about the process of consultation. To ask people for their opinion does not imply that their view will necessarily be adopted in the decision, but only that their views will be respected and taken into account. Unless this is made clear managers are likely to be accused of having already made up their minds, consulting only for 'symbolic' reasons. Not that symbolism is without its purposes.

Putting an unpopular view to a meeting of protesters may not alter the decision but at least the manager has been held to account publicly for that decision. A willingness to appear before the public in this way gradually builds a reputation for integrity which is an attribute slowly acquired but quickly lost.

Subordinates

This chapter so far has tended to assume that the manager is working at board level. Problems of accountability occur at all levels and are not made easier even where the managerial relationship is unambiguous. In what circumstances can a subordinate refuse the command of his or her superior? If a manager asks a subordinate to do something which offends that person's beliefs, such as asking a pacifist to be involved in civil defence, it is reasonable to explore how the beliefs might be acknowledged without causing difficulties in the organisation. If, however, the subordinate is critical of the manner in which it is proposed to undertake an assignment, for instance, taking a shortcut through standing orders, a healthy organisation will already have in place a grievance procedure which allows referral of the matter to a third party. It is not in the public interest for staff to be forced to act against their better judgement, but equally it is up to staff to be clear as to the basis of their objections and to be prepared to be open about them.

With professional health carers the matter is both clearer and more difficult. Codes of conduct indicate to doctors, nurses and other clinical staff what is acceptable and what is not. However, this is particularly difficult to handle when, for instance, the issue is about staffing levels. The management may feel that whatever the staffing level, the nurses' first duty is to look after their patients to the best standard they are capable of. But the nurses may claim that those standards are impossible to achieve given the workload. Ethically, the patient should receive whatever is available, sufficient or not, but it is important for nurses to have their objections recorded. It is doubtful that the public interest is served by going to the press before using the channels within the organisation, but those procedures must be available. Coercion of junior staff is unacceptable. It serves no one's interest and the protection of the more senior person by this means is unlikely to succeed except in the short term.

Conclusion

Managers in the NHS have a difficult role. At various times they are patient advocates, public representatives, government spokespersons and at all times thinking individuals. They are held responsible for the effective performance of the organisation and they are required to manage in full view of the public they serve. In this way they are in a much more exposed position than their counterparts in private industry. However, the private sector manager is accountable to the shareholders in a manner which is far less tolerant of failure and excuses than the NHS. NHS managers have to manage the ambiguities of their role and simultaneously to satisfy their immediate public, their staff and the politicians. To do this they may need to re-examine their own set of values to ensure that they are able to do what they think is right.

Managerial accountability is about demonstrating that one has tried to do the best one could according to explicit standards. But it is too much to ask that one achieve success every time.

Part two

Ray Rowden

In the wake of scandal involving alleged mismanagement in the Wessex and West Midland Regional Health Authorities, the Secretary of State established a task force to examine corporate governance in the National Health Service (DoH, 1994).

The task force published its report for consultation in January 1994. It recommends the acceptance of a clear national statement of values for the whole NHS. It proposes that this statement should act as a backdrop against which all NHS staff operate.

In addition, the task force suggests clearer rules for the appointment and conduct of chairs and non-executive directors (NEDs) on all NHS boards and suggests that all boards should have clear arrangements for declaration of any conflicts of interest and proper audit mechanisms to test the probity of board conduct.

In the post-reformed NHS, where there are concerns over the appointment of NEDs and over more business being conducted behind closed doors by unelected people, the report of the task force could go some way towards reassuring the public and NHS staff that clear standards of behaviour and conduct are to be explicitly stated and followed. The report also suggests that all NHS trusts must publish the remuneration received by all directors in their annual reports.

Health management is an increasingly broadly based profession, containing people from an increasingly wide variety of backgrounds and health service managers, unlike the clinical professions, have no regulation by statute and no professional disciplinary machinery. If a nurse or doctor practises in a manner considered dangerous to the public, the practitioner can be deregistered and will not get employment elsewhere. This is not the case for health managers, who in theory could foul up a job on a grand scale only to re-emerge in another post in another organisation, with no sanctions beyond those involving employment law.

Managers themselves have questioned this state of affairs (Stokoe, 1992) and are actively considering their position. The Institute of Health Services Management (IHSM) in the latter part of 1993 undertook an analysis of members' opinions on the issue of ethics in health management (Murray, 1993). This work exposed a complex set of issues and concerns relating to the role and functions of the manager and the ethical basis of management practice.

Following this analysis, the IHSM is undertaking in the first half of 1994 a wide-ranging consultation exercise with its 10 000 members and with external organisations with legitimate interests in health care. This external consultation is involving statutory and professional bodies, medical Royal colleges, trade unions, community health councils and a variety of consumer interests.

Arising out of this consultation, the IHSM may consider adopting a code of conduct for health managers. The Institute will certainly be organising a series of publications and educational activities to ensure that the issue of management ethics remains centre stage. While the IHSM recognises that it will not fulfil the role of a statutory body in a sector as diverse as health management, nevertheless as the leading professional organisation in health management it has recognised the need to foster debate and consider where it stands on ethical practice in the management of the health service.

Recent publicity concerning a perceived growth of bureaucracy and 'men in grey suits' makes it imperative that health managers consider their role and image far more carefully. For managers to state explicitly their adherence to ethical values and ethical behaviour is important.

Much has been made of 'whistleblowers' in the NHS. Since the NHS reforms some trusts have imposed clauses in employment contracts which make it clear that staff who venture outside the organisation with complaints could jeopardise their employment status. In truth, many NHS trusts have no such clauses in employment contracts. Some, such as West Lambeth Community Trust in London, explicitly state in their business plan that all staff are free to speak to external organisations, including the media.

Increasingly, other trusts are establishing mechanisms whereby an independent chairperson leads the oversight of investigations into serious complaints. One trust has established an independent ombudsman within the organisation. These are innovative ideas which may give NHS staff greater confidence that they can raise legitimate complaints within the organisation and have them considered by an independent and senior source.

The NHS also has a number of statutory organisations which scrutinize aspects of care and can use statutory powers to influence events or effect change.

In services for people with mental health problems and for the aged the Health Advisory Service (HAS) has a role in inspecting providers and purchasers and in promulgating good practice. HAS reports go directly to the Secretary of State in each constituent country of the United Kingdom and are public documents. HAS reports have been critical in exposing bad practice and in supporting staff who have raised legitimate complaints.

Also, in the mental health field, the Mental Health Act Commission, an independent body, is charged with ensuring that the conditions of the Mental Health Acts are complied with. The Commission has regional offices and teams which regularly monitor standards of treatment and care. All staff are free to seek advice or guidance from the Commission and to raise genuine issues of concern. The Commission can, in exceptional circumstances, accept complaints on a confidential basis.

The NHS is also covered by the Office of the Parliamentary Ombudsman, an officer who reports directly to a parliamentary select committee for administration, independent of ministers. The Commissioner has a duty to investigate all complaints of a non-clinical nature and has a full-time staff of investigating officers. The Commissioner's reports are public and are seen by the Secretary of State. The Commissioner has wide-ranging powers of investigation and recommendations from the Commissioner are rarely ignored in the service.

All NHS staff are constituents of Members of Parliament. The accountability of the Secretary of State is ultimately to Parliament. Parliament has a select committee on health affairs to provide independent scrutiny of health issues. NHS staff members can, of course, raise matters of concern with their MP, who can take matters up with ministers directly or through the Select Committee.

Whilst NHS staff have to recognise that they sometimes enter a potential minefield in raising issues of concern, it is clear that some avenues are open to them. It is also clear that government and managers are becoming increasingly concerned about issues of accountability and ethical management practice. These changes could do much to make the culture and climate of the NHS more open, more ethical and less threatening to NHS staff who wish to raise issues of concern.

References

DAVIES, P. (1991) Thumbs down for Oregon rations. *Health Service Journal* **101(5278)**, 10–11.

DAY, P. AND KLEIN, R. (1987) *Accountabilities: Five Public Services.* Tavistock, London.

DoH (1992) *Local Voices*, attached to EL92(1). Department of Health, London.

DoH (1994) *Report of Corporate Governance Task Force.* Department of Health, London.

KOONTZ, H. AND O'DONNELL, C. (1972) *Principles of Management*, 5th ed. McGraw-Hill Koyakusha, Tokyo.

MASSEY, A. (1993) *Managing the Public Sector.* Elgar, Aldershot.

MURRAY, D. J. (1993) Consultation on Management and Ethics. Unpublished paper. IHSM, London.

STARKS, M. (1991) *Not For Profit, Not For Sale.* Policy Journals, Newbury.

STOKOE, R. (1992) Presidential Address to Annual IHSM Conference. IHSM, London.

3

Medical accountability

Margaret Stacey

Introduction

For the past 135 years, British doctors have had privileged arrangements for accounting for themselves; privileged not only among other health care workers but also among all other occupations. They are also faced with a confusing array of circumstances and ways in which they may be called to account. In this chapter I shall discuss the nature of this apparent paradox, the stresses which the medical accountability system (if it can be called that) is presently subject to and suggest some ways forward. I shall also examine how difficult the majority of the population find it to bring a doctor to account when they feel aggrieved.

The notion of accountability has a long history (Day and Klein, 1987) and has meant rather different things at different times. In this chapter, following the *Oxford English Dictionary*, I am taking it to mean binding one to give an account of one's action(s), for accountability includes the notion of a necessary requirement. It means being responsible, for things or to people. A doctor may be held to account for their actions in many ways: to individual patients for clinical actions and in clinical audit to peers and colleagues; to the profession for their behaviour; to employers for the money spent and possibly also for the priorities adopted in treatments; to employers in relation to contracts and, in the NHS, ultimately to the state. Doctors, like all others, are also accountable to the civil and criminal law.

Accountability is based on legal requirements and moral expectations. Whether in the NHS or the private sector, patients consulting and receiving treatment from health care professionals should be able to trust them to be competent at their jobs; to offer the best service available, but without unnecessary interventions; not to exploit their position for their own interests, material, financial or sexual. Individually and collectively, doctors and other health care professionals should be accountable to patients for their practice in these matters.

When accountability is working properly, a patient or relative who feels these conditions have been breached is able to express the complaint or make a claim and to achieve explanation and/or redress as appropriate. Any formal system designed to this end should be universally available, equitable, accessible, as well as compassionate and humane towards both patients and professionals, recognising each as of equal worth. The contemporary arrangements for medical accountability fall short of these requirements. This chapter will argue that professional privilege, especially that of the medical profession, is an important reason for this.

The special position of doctors

Clinical autonomy and professional self-regulation

The privileged position of doctors was established in 1858 when the General Medical Council (GMC) was founded – nearly a century before the NHS. The GMC is a statutory body based on the principle of professional self-regulation achieved by the maintenance of a register of qualified medical practitioners. The principle underlying the GMC is that in return for the privilege of self-regulation the profession guarantees to ensure that the public may trust the doctors we consult – a pact made between the profession and the state (Merrison, 1975). To this end, those it registers should be fit and competent to practise.

The GMC has two prime tasks: establishing the qualifications needed for registration and ensuring that those on the register continue to be fit to practise. The first is the responsibility of the Education Committee which works closely with the medical schools; the second, of the disciplinary committees on conduct and health. The Conduct Committee investigates cases of practitioners who have been convicted of an offence in the courts or who have been referred to it as possibly being guilty of serious professional misconduct. The Health Committee examines cases of doctors who are thought to be unfit to practise by reason of health.

Within this framework the notion is that each doctor is accountable only to their individual patients and, like other citizens, to the law. This notion is associated with the doctrine of clinical autonomy whereby each doctor is solely responsible for their clinical decisions and actions. If these are questioned only peers may comment on their appropriateness. Using these doctrines, doctors successfully evaded the managerial control imposed on all other health care occupations in the 1974 NHS reorganisation, but have been unable entirely to evade the subsequent, more vigorous NHS managerial controls now imposed. The associated privilege of professional self-regulation has been sustained, however. When the regulation of the medical profession was last examined

(Merrison, 1975), the profession successfully kept the principle of professional self-regulation off the agenda. As will be seen, the principle has since been reconfirmed, again without debate.

The second accountability privilege which doctors enjoy is at law and is unique (Kennedy, 1987; Giesen and Hayes, 1992; Giesen, 1993; see also Ch. 9). British case law still sustains the notion that 'as long as the doctors act in accordance with the practice of a *responsible body of medical practitioners* they will not incur a legal obligation to compensate a disappointed patient' (Giesen, 1993, p. 3, emphasis in original). As Professor Ian Kennedy, former GMC member, has put it:

> In all other professions and walks of life, the standard of care by reference to which a person is judged is a matter for the court to determine. Expert evidence is *relevant but not determining*.
>
> (Kennedy, 1987, p. 17, emphasis in original)

The UK is becoming increasingly isolated in this position, not only from other members of the EC where the judicial systems are very different but from other parts of the Commonwealth. The key British judgement (Bolam v. Friern Barnett Hospital Management Committee), the 'Bolam test', has been rejected in both Australian and Canadian case law (Giesen, 1993; Giesen and Hayes, 1992, pp. 105–7).

Other privileges

Flowing from these privileges are others: within the NHS procedures, complaints which have a clinical component can only be dealt with by doctors. If the initial procedures do not satisfy the complainant an independent professional review (IPR) may be established. In this case the patient's complaint is heard by doctors in the respondent doctor's specialty but from another part of the country. The Health Ombudsman, or Health Service Commissioner (HSC), is someone to whom an unsatisfied patient or relative may turn when things have gone wrong about which they have not received a satisfactory explanation. However, the HSC is not allowed to investigate clinical complaints (Giddings, 1992).

Medical dominance in health care

From the mid-nineteenth century onwards, in the hospitals and later in the community, medical practitioners also established for themselves a dominant position in the division of health labour. This dominance related to opticians, nurses, midwives and other health care professions working with registered medical practitioners. In the statutory regulatory bodies medical domination was reflected in so far as the medical profession admitted no representatives of other health professions to the

GMC, while doctors claimed places as of right on the councils of other professions.

By excluding them from the privileges, the domination was also exerted over all other healing modes (nowadays referred to as complementary or alternative medicine). Other types of healers were permitted to practise so long as they did not use the term 'registered medical practitioner' and none was registered with the state. This exclusion bit hard when the NHS was established since only GMC registered practitioners could be employed there (or in any other state service).

Accountability through clinical audit

Not to be confused with managerial audit, clinical audit is professional self-regulation in the workplace. Its intention is to monitor continuously the outcomes of treatment. Under a variety of names it has been around for a long time (Devlin, 1990; Shaw, 1980). Obstetricians have audited maternal deaths since the 1930s and anaesthetists since the 1950s. More recently, CEPOD (Confidential Enquiry into Perioperative Deaths) and NCEPOD (National CEPOD) have extended the practice (Buck *et al.*, 1987; Devlin, 1990). Many areas of medicine remain uncovered, although audit has been pursued more vigorously since the government stressed its importance in *Working for Patients* (DoH, 1989). There is little knowledge of how effectively the findings are applied, although some research is beginning.

Rigorously applied, clinical audit can be an effective mode of competence control and accountability, uncovering things which are going wrong at the point of service delivery and preventing major disasters. Were it to be linked to disciplinary procedures it could increase accountability considerably. However, the profession have up till now insisted not only that the procedures and findings should be private but that no link with discipline, whether in the NHS or with the GMC, should be made.

Effect of medical status and privilege

One-to-one accountability, for so long claimed as appropriate by doctors, gives the patient inadequate protection. Few patients feel they are their doctor's social equal; even fewer that they are superior; all lack the specialist knowledge of the qualified practitioner. Although doctors may not always feel so, they are in a powerful position when treating patients. This being so, few patients feel able to call doctors to account just when they might wish to – or even to ask a doctor to explain again what was just said – as nurses asked to interpret doctors' advice will attest. Furthermore, the nineteenth century notion of one doctor treating one patient no longer applies to modern medicine. Nowadays patients are treated not by one person alone but by a team of people and their support services. Most obviously true in hospitals, this also applies to general practice: GPs rely on manifold back-up services provided by a variety of skilled personnel.

In addition, there is more to accountability than medical responsibility to individual patients, crucial though that is. There are questions of who is to be treated, what the priorities for treatment are to be, what is to be the balance of expenditure between different specialties or categories of patient. In short, there has to be some managerial responsibility. Employers, furthermore, are responsible for the performance of their employees and authorities for the service offered by the providers with whom they are in contract.

For these reasons some managerial control as well as formal complaints and claims procedures outside the doctor–patient relationship have been recognised as essential. Most doctors now accept this, although some more reluctantly than others. In contrast to the strongly held claims for professional autonomy, the NHS disciplinary and complaints procedures lack coherence. Like Topsy, they 'just growed'.

The NHS and medical accountability

Complaints

Making a complaint is one way patients or their relatives can call a doctor to account. In practice this turns out not to work terribly well (Lloyd-Bostock, 1992; Longley, 1992). No one set of procedures covers the entire NHS. Hospitals and family practitioners services have different arrangements. The former are salaried employees, while the latter contract their labour so that complaints against them are only admissible if they relate to an alleged breach of contract. In practice, of course, one complainant's experiences may span both services.

Although NHS trusts come under existing procedures there is still some lack of clarity about the way the procedures apply to them and what jurisdiction the health authority may have. That apart, procedural guidelines are applied variably from one hospital/health authority to another; this is also true in FHSAs although those guidelines appear to be tighter.

Continuing defensiveness on the part of professionals and managers can obstruct the proper handling of complaints. This is particularly true of medical practitioners and is a disadvantage of professional self-regulation, which relies on a strong sense of occupational solidarity. This defensiveness is unfortunate and reduces the effectiveness of accountability. As already mentioned, complaints with a clinical component are treated differently from others. The level of complainant satisfaction with IPR hearings is not high. All too often an impression is given that the visiting doctors are 'in league' with the alleged offender and do not treat the patient's or relative's account of the matters as being of equal worth to that of the respondent doctor.

NHS and medical discipline

NHS doctors may be called to account through a variety of official disciplinary procedures. In the worst case GPs may lose their contracts or salaried doctors their jobs. Many of the procedures are slow and cumbersome; it is not always clear which is relevant for the charge in hand. Sometimes the procedures are invoked against doctors who stand out against the system as, for example, Wendy Savage whose woman-friendly mode of obstetrics did not please her colleagues (Savage, 1986) or Helen Zeitlin who 'blew the whistle'. What is more, the procedures do not always pick up cases of malperforming, underperforming or incompetent doctors (some of them ill people). The 1993 scandals of misdiagnosis and mistreatment or failure to treat in cervical and bone cancer cases at widely separated centres and affecting thousands of patients demonstrated this all too clearly.

Medical accountability and private patients

Recent health policies have encouraged private practice. Aggrieved private patients may call their doctors to account on a one-to-one basis. Patients in private hospitals may call the hospital management to account, but are at its mercy. If neither of these routes provides satisfaction, such patients may turn to the law or to the relevant professional statutory body, such as the GMC for doctors or the UKCC for nurses. For private patients these regulatory councils may be crucial. As for the GMC, as I will argue, it is tilted towards the profession and only deals with serious complaints. Despite the unsatisfactory nature of NHS procedures it would appear the NHS patient is in a somewhat better position than the private patient.

Accountability and the law in practice

Despite the dice being loaded in favour of the profession, litigation – claims made for medical malpractice – has increased, although not yet up to US levels. This is partly attributable to the inadequacies of the GMC and of the NHS complaints procedures. For about the first 20 years of the NHS there were few lawyers competent in medical litigation and those who were were employed by health authorities. Although there are now many more firms willing to take cases on behalf of patients, potential claimants often have difficulty in finding good legal advice. AVMA (Action for Victims of Medical Accidents) has done a great deal to expose these problems and to support patients. The cost and the risks of litigation make it unequally available: only the wealthy and those poor enough to be awarded Legal Aid can afford to sue. Most of us are excluded.

For the professionals and officers of health authorities the cases are stressful, time-consuming and long drawn out. Litigation is even more stressful and time-consuming for claimants – and comes on top of existing distress. In addition, for them the result is something of a lottery as to the probability of success and the amount of damages which may be awarded. Claimants have a number of motives, but where death or disability has resulted from a medical accident, their or their dependents' requirements are for monetary compensation to afford them an income on which to live and/or to pay for necessary services.

In the long term, compensation for medical accidents (and nursing and any other health care accidents) should be separated from medical accountability and disciplinary procedures. All accidents (including medical accidents) should be compensated under Social Security arrangements, amounts depending on the severity of the injury and the resultant needs of the victim, their dependents or survivors. This mode would adequately and equitably meet financial needs without expensive and stressful legal wrangles (Ham *et al.*, 1988).

Challenges to medical privilege in accountability

There has been general dissatisfaction with medical accountability on the part of patients and their relatives which has been expressed in one way or another by all their representative bodies such as the Patients Association, Action for Victims of Medical Accidents (AVMA) and the Association of Community Health Councils for England and Wales (ACHCEW) (ACHCEW, 1989, 1990; ACHCEW/AVMA, 1992). The NHS complaints procedures have been challenged and the GMC criticised for not ensuring the competence of doctors (Robinson, 1988).

Continuing competence

Two problems have arisen with regard to competence. First, the medical schools have not kept up with the reforms which the GMC guidelines indicate, in part because of the royal colleges' control over postgraduate education and specialist training. Without agreed reforms in postgraduate education, reform of the undergraduate curriculum is constrained. Within and without the profession, there are consequent doubts as to whether British doctors are appropriately educated for the work they have to do within modern medicine.

Second, continuing competence is not adequately ensured. Doctors have to pay an annual fee to stay on the register, but the GMC has not used this as a test. The retention fee keeps a doctor's name on the register without question. More recently, but not formally in the GMC so far as I know, questions of re-registration have been mooted. The United Kingdom Central Council for Nursing, Midwifery and Health Visiting requires that those it registers submit an independently verified professional profile and re-register every three years. A similar provision is included in the Osteopaths Act 1993. Certain royal colleges are considering recertification, testing and continuing competence of holders of specialist qualifications.

As my research shows (Stacey, 1992a, 1992b), in fulfilling their disciplinary function the GMC have in practice, despite the high ethical standards and best intentions of members, tended to favour the profession over the public. The GMC has no inspectorate; it relies on reports from others about doctors' fitness. Merrison (1975: paras 256–59) recommended the establishment of an inhouse unit to investigate allegations against doctors: this has never been established. The profession's assurance of the continuing competence of doctors which the GMC registers has proved unreliable.

The GMC's problem in dealing with competence derives from the principle of clinical autonomy and the presumed equality of all registered doctors. Until the last 10 or 12 years the GMC only disciplined doctors for clinical failures in the grossest cases. In the past decade more have been forwarded to the Conduct Committee. However, my research (Stacey, 1992b, pp. 160–6) showed that not only did committees have difficulty finding guilt in such cases but, when found guilty, the doctors appeared to be dealt with leniently in comparison with those who had committed other offences.

A challenge reached the House of Commons 10 years ago. Nigel Spearing MP felt the the GMC procedures were inadequate to deal with a case in his constituency involving the death of a child, Alfie, the mascot of the West Ham United football team. The doctor had failed properly to treat or refer. The GMC's Conduct Committee, however, did not find this sufficiently serious to affect the doctor's registration. Spearing consequently proposed an amendment to the Medical Act which would have had the effect of introducing a second offence of 'unacceptable professional conduct' in addition to 'serious professional misconduct'. The GMC could not accept this and have spent the better part of a decade working on a way of ensuring continuing competence, which it now prefers to call 'performance', proposing a third arm to its disciplinary powers, called 'performance procedures'. These proposals also show bias to the profession (Stacey, 1992c, 1993).

Members of the public who complain to the GMC about the behaviour of a practitioner encounter a number of problems. To start with, if a patient or relative decides to complain, generally speaking they think the matter is serious, but relatively few complaints received are of a kind the GMC feels able to deal with. Between 1st September 1991 and 31st August 1992, of 1300 complaints and information considered by Council, no action was taken on 765 (rising 60%). This occurs because the GMC can only deal with complaints which call a doctor's registration into question, that is, which affect the doctor's livelihood; the matters must be 'serious'. A problem arises because what a patient may consider 'serious' the GMC screener may not: medical and lay definitions can and do differ. In the dominantly medical ethos of the Council, the recent inclusion of lay screeners has apparently not as yet given effective expression to these differences.

Of the complaints on which action is taken, few proceed to the Conduct Committee. Less than 10% went to preliminary proceedings, 2.6% to conduct and 1.8% to health (on the grounds that the doctor's fitness to practise may be impaired by reason of health – most often drink or drugs). The remainder (85%) of cases received that year were either still under consideration or had been dealt with informally.

The public tend to see the GMC as the apex of the complaints machinery. It is not that. Its statutory task is to see that doctors on the register are fit to practise. Complaints about particular doctors are seen only in that light, which the GMC defines narrowly. It is, after all, a serious matter to take away a person's livelihood, which erasure from the register does. 'There, but for the grace of God, go I' is constantly in the mind of practitioners testing a case.

Ministerial enquiries

The government has called for further investigation on a number of these issues, in part because of the major changes in the NHS, in part because of professional and public disquiet. A committee under Professor Wilson, Vice Chancellor of Leeds University, was established in the summer of 1993 to review the NHS complaints procedures. Let us hope that this review faces up to the many outstanding problems, including those flowing from special medical pleading. Let us also hope that, although complaints to the GMC lie outside the committee's terms of reference, it examines carefully the interrelationship between the GMC's procedures and those of the NHS. A problem has been that the

NHS procedures and the regulatory body's procedures have always been treated separately. It has become urgent to look at them together if the effectiveness of medical accountability is to be properly assessed.

The scandals regarding apparently incompetent NHS hospital doctors mentioned earlier led the government in the autumn of 1993 to establish another committee under Sir Kenneth Calman, the Chief Medical Officer for England (CMO) to 'review current guidance and procedures relating to doctors whose performance appears to fall below acceptable standards . . . to make recommendations . . . for any necessary changes and further work needed'. In November 1992 the GMC had asked the government to make Parliamentary time available for legislation to extend its disciplinary powers to include performance procedures. By the time the Calman Committee was established, this had not been done. Was this just because of shortage of time or is there perhaps a major rethink going on?

In addition to proposing these procedures, the GMC intend to increase the proportion of lay members to something like a fifth of the Council. This will help to establish a more independent lay voice; lay members will at least be able to consult among each other and exchange a range of views. However, the absence of a constituency for them to turn to – in contrast to the medical members who can refer to the BMA or their medical school or royal college – will continue to be a problem. Habits of deference die hard. These proposals may be seen as another example of the GMC belatedly attempting to reform itself before it has its reforming done for it, without perhaps fully realising the radical extent of the changes that are needed. Undoubtedly many members are acutely aware of the seriousness of present challenges. They worry about the status of medicine but are also greatly concerned that medicine shall offer a good and reliable service.

Richard Smith, editor of the *British Medical Journal*, clearly fears it may be too late. Writing soon after the Calman review was announced, his leader 'The end of the GMC?' caused anger in the Council. Smith (1993) noted that it seemed the GMC was being 'sidelined'. Certainly, a whole series of events can be read as adding up to that conclusion. Hitherto when challenged the medical establishment has been remarkably skilful at compromising just enough to retain most of its power and privileges. Will it succeed this time?

Pros and cons of self-regulation

Does the problem lie in self-regulation itself or the form it has taken in the GMC and royal colleges? Self-regulation may be defended on the ground that rulings from peers are more salient and better accepted than from outsiders. 'Closing ranks' could take even more serious forms, amounting perhaps to 'ganging up', if investigations were seen as attacks by outsiders. This could be true of any occupation, let alone one with the historical past of medicine.

Not enough is known about various regulatory mechanisms and their effects. However, my research suggests professional self-regulation will always be likely to favour the profession over the public. Under this arrangement the regulatory body, if it is to do its task, has to retain the support and maintain the unity of the profession. At the workplace doctors, like others, are reluctant to 'shop' colleagues. This tendency for the GMC to favour the profession has not been weakened by the 1979 Act which gave elected medical members a majority on the Council. Yet to the rank and file of doctors the GMC is remote: many feel alienated.

Nevertheless, there is a strong case for having a well-organised and united medical profession (body of professional workers) independent of the state, not only in the interests of the profession itself but to speak up for the health of the nation from the point of view of skilled independent knowledge. An example is the BMA's report on the effects of the 'care in the community' policy which GPs say in their experience has not improved the care which their elderly patients are receiving (*The Independent*, 25.11.93). The centralising tendency of the governments of the last 14 years, which has weakened universities, schools, local government and the trade unions, has underlined this need. Furthermore, the great majority of British doctors provide a good and reliable service. Procedures are needed for the incompetent or careless minority.

Professional self-regulation confirmed?

Recent legislation has given greater autonomy to some other health care occupations, notably nurses, midwives and health visitors through the Nurses, Midwives and Health Visitors Acts 1979 and 1992. Osteopaths are now to be state registered (Osteopaths Act 1993). The medical profession supported these developments. Former GMC President Lord Walton played a supportive role in the passage of the 1992 Act for nursing and a prominent one in proposing the first Osteopaths Bill. In the debates fresh confirmation was given to the principle of professional self-regulation, again without it being examined, notably by Lord Ennals, Earl Baldwin of Bewdley and Lord Carter (Hansard, 31.1.91, Vol. 534, pp. 1598, 1600, 1609). Paradoxically, there is reason to doubt whether self-regulation for complementary medicines is necessarily the best route for them or the public (Stacey, in press).

By agreeing to the extension of self-regulation to selected complementary practices the leaders of the medical profession have both retained self-regulation and the dominance of biomedicine in the health care division of labour; under the Act, for example, osteopaths may not practise in the NHS, but only privately. These developments have been supported by the very government which has established the Wilson and Calman reviews.

Either the government has not given due thought to the problems or is pursuing a tacit policy of tightening professional self-regulation without overtly examining it. Regular performance review and re-registration is provided in the Acts for nursing and osteopathy. This could be extended, as could regular reporting to Parliament. Such an opportunistic and tacit policy (if such it is) has the grave disadvantage that the principle of self-regulation and what checks there should be on it are not publicly discussed or analysed. Perhaps the Calman review will discuss this and open up its thinking for public discussion.

Which way is forward?

Given all the possible routes and the difficulty of getting information about them, citizens who want to call doctors to account find themselves in a jungle with no clearly marked pathways. Complainants have no one way into the confusing array of procedures. Furthermore, it is nobody's business to look at medical accountability in the round.

The most radical proposal afoot is to create a Health Standards Inspectorate (HSI) for all health professions, as AVMA and ACHCEW (ACHCEW/AVMA, 1992) suggest, replacing all existing bodies. It would cover all aspects of health and all types of professionals and workers. It would aim to ensure continuing competence of practitioners, managers and service provision and would replace existing NHS complaints machinery. While possibly too radical to be politically feasible, the proposal merits careful attention, for the issues it raises need to be addressed by any reform which is likely to be effective.

I have argued (Stacey, 1992b, pp. 259–70), perhaps idealistically, that medicine should transform itself and ask for the GMC to be turned into a council under lay control including, as well as doctors, other health care professionals as of right. At present there are few signs of any such radical move.

Whatever else happens, members of the public who wish to call a doctor to account should have available to them an easily accessible sympathetic office where they can go with their complaint and be directed to the most appropriate part of the accountability process. The other essential is that at the highest level there should be a body with overall responsibility to see that medical accountability is working properly, covering NHS and private practice and professional as well as NHS regulatory bodies.

Various proposals have been made: a council overseeing all the professions (Klein, 1973, pp. 160–3); such a council but for the health professions only; the HSC to be given oversight of the GMC as well as the NHS, private as well as NHS patients, with freedom to enquire into clinical complaints. The disadvantage of the first two ideas is that they imply yet another quango. Its annual answerability to Parliament would be essential as well as accountability of the members to some sort of public constituency. There is not space here to develop these ideas in any detail, but they are among those which should be discussed. For most but not all doctors, any of these ideas are unwelcome.

Conclusion

A thoroughgoing and open discussion about the value of professional self-regulation is needed. Issues in medical accountability are complex because of the outdated historical baggage which is carried, because of the complexity of the system and the many skilled workers involved and because of the inherently delicate nature of the tasks to be accounted for.

Claims are made that medicine is a very special occupation and that as well as the technical skills provided there is something magical or sacred in the doctor–patient relationship. Be that as it may, it is clear that patients need to be able to trust doctors. Medicine (like nursing and other health care professions) is clearly special in that the patient is, paradoxically, part of the workforce – an unpaid health worker. In a free society no treatment can proceed without the patient's cooperation; in some treatments a great deal of activity is required from the patient, for example, in stoma care or home renal dialysis.

This is the special nature of medicine to which attention must be paid in designing accountability procedures. To meet the criteria enunciated at the outset, appropriate space and dignity should be offered to patients and their representatives as well as to potential patients, that is the public at large. Whatever interim measures are designed to improve accountability in the short term, this implies that eventually the final arbiter in the medical accountability process should be a lay body served by medical practitioners as the technically skilled workers. Within that ultimate boundary there would be space for self-regulation, but it would best be undertaken by a medical profession which, as I have suggested elsewhere (Stacey, 1992b, Ch. 17), had espoused a new kind of professionalism, in which service was the first priority and in which other health workers and patients were recognised as members of the health team having equal worth.

Acknowledgements

My gratitude to the Leverhulme Emeritus Fellowship which has made it possible for me to continue my research on the GMC, begun with an ESRC grant (GOO 232247); to Dr Phil Moss for his research help for this chapter; and to Jennifer Lorch for her continued support. What is written here is, however, my responsibility alone.

References

ACHCEW (1989) *NHS Complaints Procedures: A Report of a Conference held 11.10.88.* Association of Community Health Councils for England and Wales, London.

ACHCEW (1990) *National Health Service Complaints Procedures.* Association of Community Health Councils for England and Wales, London.

ACHCEW/AVMA (1992) *A Health Standards Inspectorate.* Association of Community Health Councils for England and Wales and Action for Victims of Medical Accidents, London.

BUCK, N., DEVLIN, H. B. AND LUNN, I. N. (1987) *The Report of a Confidential Enquiry into Perioperative Deaths.* Nuffield Provincial Hospitals Trust and King's Fund, London.

DAY, P. AND KLEIN, R. (1987) *Accountabilities: Five Public Services.* Tavistock, London.

DoH (1989) *Working for Patients.* HMSO, London.

DEVLIN, H. B. (1990) Audit and the quality of clinical care. *Annals of the Royal College of Surgeons of England* 1, 3–14 (Suppl.)

GIDDINGS, P. (1992) Complaints, Remedies and the Health Service Commissioner, Paper presented to the 1992 Political Studies Association Conference, The Queen's University, Belfast. The University of Reading Centre for Ombudsman Studies, Reading.

GIESEN, D. (1993) Legal accountability for the provision of medical care: a comparative view. *Journal of the Royal Society of Medicine* **86(11)**, 648–52.

GIESEN, D. AND HAYES, J. (1992) The patient's right to know – a comparative view. *Anglo-American Law Review* **21(2)**, 101–22.

HAM, C., DINGWALL, R., FENN, P. and HARRIS, D. (1988) *Medical Negligence: Compensation and Accountability.* King's Fund Institute, London.

KENNEDY, I. (1987) Review of the year 2: confidentiality, competence and malpractice. In *Medicine in Contemporary Society: King's College Studies 1986–7*, P. Byrne (ed.), pp. 49–63. King's College Hospital Fund for London, London.

KLEIN, R. (1973) *Complaints Against Doctors: A Study in Professional Accountability.* Charles Knight, London.

LLOYD-BOSTOCK, S. (1992) Attributions and apologies in letters of complaint to hospitals and letters of response. In *Attributions, Accounts and Close Relationships*, J. H. Harvey, T. Orburk and A. Weber (eds), pp. 209–20. Springer-Verlag, Berlin.

LONGLEY, D. (1992) Out of order. *Health Service Journal* **102** (**5330**), 22–4.

LONGLEY, D. (1993) *Public Law and Health Service Accountability.* Open University Press, Buckingham.

MERRISON, A. (1975) *Report of the Committee of Enquiry into the Regulation of the Medical Profession.* Cmnd 6018. HMSO, London.

ROBINSON, J. (1988) *A Patient Voice at the GMC: A Lay Member's View of the General Medical Council.* Health Rights Report No. 1, London.

SAVAGE, W. (1986) *A Savage Enquiry.* Virago, London.

SHAW, C. D. (1980) Acceptability of audit. *British Medical Journal* **281**, 1443–5.

SMITH, R. (1993) The end of the GMC? *British Medical Journal* **307**, 954.

STACEY, M. (1992a) Medical accountability: a background paper. In *Challenges in Medical Care*, A. Grubb (ed.), pp. 109–39. Wiley, Chichester.

STACEY, M. (1992b) *Regulating British Medicine: The General Medical Council.* Wiley, Chichester.

STACEY, M. (1992c) For public or profession? The new GMC performance procedures. *British Medical Journal* **305**, 1085–7.

STACEY, M. (1993) Green shoots: the new GMC proposals. *Health Service Journal* **103** (**5336**), 20–22.

STACEY, M. (1994) Collective therapeutic responsibility; lessons from the GMC. In *The Healing Bond*, S. Budd and U. Sharma (eds) Routledge, London.

4

Nursing accountability

Jean Orr

Accountability has become an increasingly important issue in nursing. Many writers and commentators see accountability as a fundamental attribute of any occupation that wishes to become a profession. Accountability, in the sense of being answerable for one's behaviour and actions, is now seen as necessary and desirable for autonomous nursing practice.

There are many issues involved in how accountability is perceived and practised by the 600 000 nurses, midwives and health visitors who are registered with the United Kingdom Central Council (UKCC), the statutory body which regulates the three professions. Any debate about accountability in nursing must include an examination of the role of the UKCC and the efforts it has made in highlighting the importance of nurses being accountable for their own practice.

The UKCC – setting the standard

The UKCC was established by the Nurses, Midwives and Health Visitors Act in 1979 and was charged with the major function of maintaining and improving standards of training and professional conduct. Two thirds of the Council's membership is elected by the profession and the remaining one third is appointed by the Department of Health to represent academic, medical and lay interests. Early in its life, the first Council set about drawing up a Code of Professional Conduct (UKCC, 1992a) which set out the standards required of practitioners on the Council's register. The Code, which is regularly renewed to take account of health care systems and case law arising out of professional conduct hearings, is in its third edition. It is regarded by the majority of the profession as the benchmark against which to measure practice and a means of heightening awareness and understanding of what being an accountable practitioner means. The Code, in its introductory clause, states that practitioners are accountable at all times, whether engaged in current

practice or not and whether on or off duty. In situations where the practitioner is employed they will be accountable to the employer for providing service which they are employed to provide and for the proper use of resources made available by the employer for the purpose. The practitioner is ultimately accountable to the UKCC for any failure to satisfy the requirements of this introductory paragraph of the Code. Therefore, accountability is seen as an integral part of professional practice, since in the course of that practice the practitioner has to make judgements in a wide variety of circumstances and be answerable for those judgements.

The Code seeks to state important principles which should guide practice. The interests of the public and the patient or client are seen as paramount and the practitioner should recognise that these interests must predominate over those of the nurse. In addition, each practitioner must be personally and professionally accountable in such a manner as to respect the primacy of the interests of the client.

The UKCC has produced a number of advisory documents which elaborate upon and supplement the Code of Professional Conduct, one of which is entitled *Exercising Accountability* (UKCC, 1989). Dimond (1989), in reviewing this document, congratulates the UKCC on providing practitioners with detailed guidelines for the many situations of conflict they face. In particular, she refers to the emphasis on the importance of the responsibility and duties that nurses have when there are shortcomings in the environment of care and when it is apparent that patients have not fully understood the implications of consenting to a specific treatment or have not been given the information they need about their condition. In addition, the document highlights the nurse's role where a patient requires an advocate and where there are problems in relation to collaboration and co-operation in care.

Reg Pyne, the UKCC's Assistant Registrar for Standards and Ethics, has been a leading writer and campaigner on the accountability issue (Pyne, 1992b). He sees the UKCC's documents as part of the means by which nursing is being changed from an occupation which traditionally regarded good conduct as primarily being compliant and submissive into a profession which now regards good conduct as primarily being honest, responsible, questioning and challenging. This is necessary because these are the qualities which, together with knowledge and skills, best serve the interests of patients and clients. According to Pyne, far too many practitioners still do not properly understand their personal and professional accountability and do not recognise their own vulnerability. He argues that they allow themselves to be lulled into slack practices which create risks for patients and cast aside good standards. They allow themselves to be persuaded into accepting delegated tasks beyond their competence and have not yet developed a knowledge base sufficient to question and challenge. He maintains that blind, unthinking and

unquestioning obedience and refusal to challenge anything exposes patients to risk. The following case illustrates my point.

Case Study 1

Two young registered nurses employed in a paediatric unit became concerned when two consultant anaesthetists were seen to be prescribing drugs for premedication for children which were far in excess of anything previously prescribed for the purpose. Having first spoken to the ward sister and discovering that she shared their concern but did not believe it to be her place to question the doctors, they raised their concerns with the anaesthetists and were told by them that they were engaged in a research project, that it would be all right and that they, the anaesthetists, would bear the full responsibility.

Still concerned, realising from the manufacturer's literature that the quantities being prescribed were often 10 or more times the recommended maximum dose (for children of the body weight involved), the nurses (through one of their number) telephoned the manufacturers. The technical spokesman of the firm expressed his horror at what he had been told, but declined to confirm his concern in writing.

Enquiries which the nurses directed to the nurse member of the local ethical committee revealed that no such research project had been before the committee for approval.

The nurses, having tested their concerns as described, bluntly told the anaesthetists that they knew they had been deceived and that, while it was for the doctors to prescribe what they wished, they (the nurses) would not administer doses such as those prescribed. Further to that, they would feel it necessary to make a record of their reasons and would contemplate informing the parents of any children for whom such excessive doses were prescribed without consent. There was a sudden return to orthodox prescribing.

Accountability and practice

While health authorities have been formulating policies and practices for nurses, the debate about accountability has only recently come to the attention of most nurses, following the development of the Code of Professional Conduct. There was a general belief among nurses that they

were 'covered' in some way by employers or doctors. There was confusion between the notion of professional responsibility and legal cover in an employment context. This was most probably due to a lack of clear professional guidelines and lack of knowledge about contractor requirements as well as the imbalance of power in the relationship between nurses and doctors and between senior nurses and junior nurses.

In the past, nurses were used to carrying out doctors' orders and some did not see themselves as accountable beyond that task. Nurses were often placed in difficult situations when asked to act on doctors' orders while being concerned about what they were being asked to do. For example, it was common practice on night duty for a nurse to phone the doctor on call if a patient was in pain and ask for medication to be authorised. The nurse knew that the drugs should be written up in the patient's notes before being given but was often told to give the drug on the understanding that the doctor would write it up in the morning. Many similar situations existed in nursing where there was a tension between wanting to help the doctor and alleviating the plight of the patient. Although the hospital's policies forbade such activities, there was an expectation that the nurse would 'help the doctor' and consequently help the patient. Within the hierarchial structure of hospitals, it is all too easy to see how nurses could find themselves facing dilemmas such as this in the course of their work.

Thompson *et al.* (1988) point out that nurses have a duty to the profession to behave in a manner which upholds codes of conduct, even though the organisation within which they work gives more weight to doctors' opinions. They go on to say that nurses must be responsible for the care they give and cannot claim that working to doctors' orders makes them exempt from any responsibility. For example, if a nurse thinks a prescription contains the wrong dose they have the duty to question this and if there still is a doubt they have a duty to refuse to give it. This of course requires knowledge and assertiveness.

To illustrate this point, I will draw on the experience of an American colleague who, while undertaking research in a UK hospital, was asked to give a drug to a very ill patient. She looked at the notes, studied the laboratory reports and refused to give the drug as she believed it would kill the patient. The junior hospital doctor told her to give it and she refused. She telephoned the registrar who also told her to give it. She again refused and telephoned the consultant at home on a Sunday morning. This was a grave action as the consultant was known to be 'difficult'. When she stated her concerns, he said she was quite right not to give the drug. This colleague happened to be the author of a major American text book on pharmacology and knew what she was talking about. What about the average nurse who would not have the level of assertiveness and knowledge to ensure that the patient was not harmed? The nurses on the ward in which my colleague worked were unsupportive of her actions. Her challenge to medical domination was seen as a threat to them as it showed up their lack of knowledge and challenged the status quo. This nurse had come from a very different background in which nurses do not see themselves as subordinate to doctors. Many American nurses have an education to Masters degree and doctoral level and are in a better position to demonstrate accountability for the care given.

From this example, we can see two major problems in the area of accountability. Firstly, the nurse has to have confidence in her own worth as a nurse and all that this means for her responsibility for care. Secondly, she has to have the knowledge to back up her actions. This involves having the support of the profession so that her actions to protect the patients are acceptable. One could ask why nurses feel unable to act at all times to protect patients and one reason may be that nursing management is not as supportive as it should and could be. It has to be said that nurses in the past have not been seen to speak out about concerns regarding patient care and other health service matters. But cutbacks in the service and the changing ideology, which can be seen to threaten standards of care, have made it imperative that they have the freedom to do so. It could be that in the past there was less emphasis on speaking out because of a belief that the service was always operating in the best interests of patients. Current government changes are so threatening that many nurses now realise the dangers to the service and to the patient. Nurses are recognising their responsibility for the care they give, due to the increased emphasis on accountability by the UKCC and the publicity given to its disciplinary procedures. Nurses are increasingly worried about being reported to the UKCC for failure to carry out care of a sufficient and acceptable standard.

Pyne says that nurses coming before the professional conduct hearings of the UKCC often demonstrate a lack of awareness about who they are accountable to. In response to the question 'To whom are you accountable?', the nurse may name the health authority, the government, David Hunt, Virginia Bottomley, the Prime Minister, the UKCC and the doctor, all before the patient, if indeed the patient features on the list at all. On the rare occasions that patients are mentioned first, the answer is probably given by a student nurse or by someone still within three or four months of initial registration. Pyne says that the further the nurse moves away from initial registration, the more distorted the understanding of accountability becomes. This is despite the fact that in the 14 clauses of the Code of Professional Conduct patients are directly mentioned in seven and are the rationale behind the others. Furthermore, the Code warns registered practitioners that they are accountable for their practice, not someone else acting as proxy, and that they are personally accountable for what they do, for what they fail to do and for what happens within their sphere of influence.

Power relations in the NHS

It is inadequate to discuss the issue of accountability without setting it in the context of the power relations which exist in the health service. This power not only rests on status or the balance of status between one professional group and another but also on gender. There are many parallels between the role of nurses, of which 90% are women, and the role of women in society. Women have the traditional role of protecting the privacy of the family and the man in particular. Frequently women are expected to collude in the silences and secrecy of the home and this can be translated into the hospital situation where nurses frequently know much more than they may ever disclose. There is very little research in this area as it is such a hidden and accepted feature of the nursing world. However, in talking to nurses, it is clear that the norm is to support the system and the doctors as the most powerful group within that system. Nurses have also colluded in some situations with other nurses, particularly in closed institutions such as in the mental illness and mental handicap field.

The status of an employee, such as a nurse, raises questions about the relationship between accountability to the organisation and accountability to the patient. The nurse is contracted to follow the policies, rules and regulations of the organisation and must be accountable to that organisation and management structure for carrying out the organisational function. This is not as clearcut as it might seem. One might assume that the goals and aims of the organisation in terms of health care would be consistent with the standard and improvement of patient care. However, this may not always be the case. Part of the confusion is the lack of clear role boundaries between what is nursing work and what is medical work. There can sometimes be tension between the professional ethos of nurses, with their ability to make direct and independent decisions in the nursing care of patients, and the views of others in the organisation. The independent decision making of the nurse may not be seen as legitimate by her superiors or by medical colleagues. With increasing skill mix on the wards and fewer trained staff, nurses may be asked to undertake tasks and accept responsibility in excess of their knowledge base and experience. There is a difficulty in nurses being accountable as a group when they are not a homogeneous group. Nurses are educationally diverse, ranging from the enrolled nurse with two years preparation to the nurse with a registered qualification and educational preparation to primary, masters or doctoral degree level. It is often difficult, therefore, for patients and colleagues to understand that nurses are not equal in terms of education and in what they might reasonably be expected to do. This may also limit the organisation's willingness to allow autonomy of nursing practice to be extended to all nurses.

With the dilution of skilled nursing care in most settings, nurses are being expected to supervise and be accountable for the care given by non-nurse workers such as health care assistants. Certainly, nurses are instructed to delegate tasks to others only when they are sure of the other's ability. But how is this to be judged in a busy ward or isolated community setting? Delegation will pose additional strain and responsibility on registered nurses. Consider the following case.

Case Study 2

The combination of limited financial resources and increasing problems of recruitment of registered nurses has led a health authority to conduct a reappraisal of its policies for staffing at night.

One of the decisions announced is that, when the operating theatres are not in action during the night, the theatre nursing staff will be redeployed. The reaction of the theatre staff to this is not to be particularly worried, since in this large city general hospital the operating theatres are busy almost every night and, if they were allocated elsewhere, they would always be placed in support of other staff as the prospect would always exist of their recall to theatre if emergencies arose. They simply stated their expectation on this point to their managers and were told nothing to disillusion them.

Some weeks later, quite exceptionally, the operating theatre was not in action three hours into the night shift. The senior staff nurse on theatre duty was suddenly instructed to go to take charge of a large, busy paediatric ward in which there were a number of very ill children. She was told by the night sister that the unqualified staff on the ward would tell her about the patients as she did not have time to go to the ward herself.

Although she has been a registered nurse for 12 years the theatre staff nurse has worked only in operating theatres for all of those 12 years. She has had no ward experience since registration and had only an eight week allocation to a paediatric ward when a student nurse.

As a first move the nurse refused to go, stating to the night sister that it would be dangerous. She cited Clause 4 of the Code of Professional Conduct and was unimpressed by the night sister telling her there was nobody else to go. The night sister called the night nursing officer to speak to the nurse. She repeated the demand, but supplemented it with some emotional blackmail statements about the poor children in danger. Initially the nurse asked why one of the night sisters was not covering the ward in that case and repeated her refusal.

After further pressure from her two superiors she said that she would go to the ward, but only after she had sat and written a document stating all the reasons why she felt it to be wrong. She said she would give one copy to the nursing officer, send one to the general manager and keep the third herself in case there were any long term repercussions of the events of the night. Then she went. Three hours later there was a rush of emergency admissions and the nurse was recalled to the operating theatre.

Education and practice

In order for nurses to be accountable for care in a professional sense, they have a duty to inform themselves of advances in the knowledge of nursing care. The profession must ensure that not only are nurses being educated to a sufficient level but that established practitioners have the motivation and facilities to get regular updating and continue their education. The UKCC has put forward recommendations for postregistration education and practice which include five study days every three years for practising nurses and the requirement that nurses returning to practice undertake an appropriate course. To date it is not clear whether employers and/or the government will be prepared to fund these initiatives or indeed give nurses time off to undertake the preparation. The costs of not doing so are high in terms of patient care. At a recent UKCC professional conduct hearing a nurse was struck off the register for misconduct in caring for vulnerable, elderly patients. He had been given employment in a private nursing home, despite the fact that he had not nursed for over 30 years. He was offered no retraining or return to practice course, yet he was in charge of the home by virtue of his registration. It could be argued that he had no right to be in this position of responsibility. The matron of the home, on the other hand, had a responsibility to her patients which she neglected.

Nurses, midwives and health visitors form the major workforce of the National Health Service and cost about £5 billion in salary costs. How they carry out their work clearly has major implications for patient care and yet very few resources are devoted to research and development of their function. This had resulted in nursing activity often being based on custom and practice rather than on relevant research findings.

It is important that nurses take on board the research findings that are available to evaluate the care that they give and to provide support for present practice. When there are rapid changes in both policy and practice new developments and innovations must be shown to be valid and seen to be improving the quality of patient care. Nurses must pay attention to empirical evidence to support their work. Much nursing in the past has been based on tradition and ritual. This is increasingly being challenged and nurses are having to defend their actions by calling on research evidence. Indeed, if the care received by the patient or client is based on tradition alone and is contrary to research findings then the patient is not being offered the best possible care and the nurse is accountable for the low standard of care that is being given.

The implementation of Project 2000, a new preparation for practice, should go some way to encouraging a thinking and critical practitioner and the increasing integration of nursing into the higher education sector should break down the monolithic approach that existed in many colleges of nursing. But of course, the effect of having nurses who are questioning and challenging will not be comfortable for those who wish to maintain the status quo. It has been a difficult struggle to implement these changes in nursing education because nursing has traditionally been seen as women's work and therefore not requiring education at university level. Indeed, within the profession itself there is often a reluctance to see educational qualifications as worthwhile and frequently there is a reticence about appearing to ask for too much. Hence we have a situation in which Project 2000 preparation is at diploma level rather than degree level, as it was felt that the latter would be demanding too much.

Accountability in the reformed health service

There are increasing barriers to accountability in large areas of the National Health Service because of 'commercial confidentiality'. The National Health Service now operates in a purchaser/provider mode and trusts are in competition with each other for resources and for selling services and there is an increasing emphasis on secrecy within their management and operation. This secrecy leads to a lack of debate in the public arena about the standards of care and impedes the sharing of good practice about patient care.

When talking to practitioners, there seems to me to be an increasing fear about speaking out regarding patients' well-being. This secrecy is sometimes taken to quite ridiculous lengths. At a recent conference, two health visitors told me that they could not make comments publicly in the conference hall as their manager was present. This manager had disciplined a colleague at a previous conference for speaking out about what was happening in their area. It is difficult to see what is so commercially important about baby clinics and visiting services for families, although no doubt managers are sensitive to news that services are being cut or reduced.

A recent survey of health correspondents in regional daily newspapers and specialist nursing and medical magazines carried out by the union, Manufacturing Science Finance (MSF), found:

1. a climate of intimidation and fear with 71% of correspondents reporting fear of losing their job as the main reason why NHS staff would not speak out on the record;
2. a worsening situation since the NHS reforms, particularly in trusts. 85% of correspondents said the situation was worse than two years ago and 60% said staff in trusts were less likely to speak out than those in directly managed units;
3. an increase in 'gagging' clauses and policies; 71% said they were now more common than two years previously.

(Health Visitor, 1993)

The MSF report went on to call for the right of all NHS staff to go to an external authority, either the local community health council or the health ombudsman, if their employer failed to respond adequately to their concerns. MSF has set out charter values, laying down the rights and duties of NHS staff to protect and maintain standards. There is a concern that current official guidance from the Department of Health on freedom of speech in the NHS puts nurses and health visitors in breach of their common law duty of care and in breach of the UKCC Code of Professional Conduct (see Ch. 10).

As a result of the concern of nurses about the changes in the NHS and their effects on standards of care the UKCC (1992b) put out a Registrar's letter, 'The Council's Standards for Incorporation into Contracts for Hospital and Community Health Care Services'. The Council recommends that the Code of Professional Conduct and other documents such as *The Scope of Professional Practice* and *Exercising Accountability* should influence contracts between purchasers and providers of health care in the following ways:

- Purchasers should require recognition of the Code by the inclusion in contracts of employment for nurses, midwives and health visitors of a clause requiring compliance with its contents. Providers should respond positively to this requirement and be able to demonstrate to the satisfaction of the purchaser their commitment to the Code of Professional Conduct and their intention to facilitate nurses employed by them to satisfy its requirements in all aspects.
- Providers should recognise and honour the individual practitioner's right of freedom of speech, consistent with guidance issued by the government health departments.
- With regard to education and competence for continuing practice, purchasers should require providers to ensure the provision of and/or access to adequate educational opportunities for registered nurses, midwives and health visitors in order to assist them to

maintain and improve their knowledge and competencies. Providers should respond positively to this requirement by providing a skill mix relevant to the needs and interests of their patients and clients, ensuring appropriate support for newly registered practitioners and those returning to practice and honouring the UKCC requirement that each individual practitioner has at least five days leave for professional development study in any three years.

- Purchasers should require providers to have effective systems for checking with Council the registration status of all employees and to ensure that all such employees maintain effective registration. Providers should make full use of the Council's confirmation service which holds this information. They therefore avoid the risk of employing people recently removed from the register and help to identify those who purport to be registered when they are not.

- Purchasers should require providers to ensure that registered nurses, midwives and health visitors remain accountable for assessment, planning, implementation and standards of nursing, midwifery and health visiting care, even though they may delegate some aspects of such care to directly accountable support staff and providers should ensure that such support workers always work under the supervision of registered practitioners.

It is too early at this stage to say how effective the UKCC's guidelines will be and whether or not purchasers and providers will pay any attention to the document. The UKCC routinely informs health authorities about cases of professional misconduct in their areas and, on occasion, transcripts of the full proceedings of professional conduct hearings have been sent to regional chairpersons of the health authorities in which the practitioner was employed. This information will now be sent to those who purchase the service from the trust in which the nurse is employed. This may very well have a powerful effect on standards of care as, in many instances, although the individual practitioner may have been at fault, the overriding environment in which misconduct took place is such that important questions would be raised for the management and organization of the service. One presumes that purchasers will only want to buy services from areas where the standard of care is good.

This is all very well in theory. However, there may be a dilemma for practitioners in respect of the environment of care and this is becoming an increasing area for concern with shortfalls in service, reduction in staffing and changes in skill mix. It is difficult for nurses to speak out for fear of losing their jobs, particularly if they are on short term contracts and where there is an oversupply of nurses. This is a particularly difficult area, as we have seen, for those nurses and doctors who have blown the whistle and whose careers have suffered as a result. However, the UKCC is adamant that nurses ought to be reporting shortfalls in service and other factors that could jeopardise standards of care and safety of patients. The following case illustrates the kind of thing which can be achieved.

Case Study 3

A nurse was newly appointed to a post as the nursing officer for a neurosurgical unit of three wards. Almost immediately she observed that, on all the wards in the unit, although the trained nursing staff was adequate, all the major nursing care, including such activities as neurological observations and the care of patients newly admitted with cranial injuries, was performed by unqualified staff working unsupervised.

Concerned at what she regarded as completely unnecessary and improper delegation, the new nursing officer raised the matter in a meeting with all the ward sisters (all of whom had been in post for a substantial period of time) and was surprised that the reaction she received from them was first to state that they could see nothing wrong and second to point out that the previous nursing officer knew all about it and that her superiors had demonstrated confidence in her by promoting her. Disturbed by this reaction, the nursing officer sought to raise the matter at a higher level, only to receive a fairly similar response.

Being determined to find a genuine solution to the problem rather than an expedient response, the nurse arrived at a decision. Rather than ask her managers what she should do, she declared to them what she was going to do. She indicated that she was personally going to conduct a review of work and working practices in the unit over a period of several weeks and that she would spend time with all members of staff on all wards and shifts. She provided for her managers the terms of reference she had set herself for the review and stated the date on which she would provide a report complete with decisions and/or recommendations.

Her review showed that her cause for concern was well-founded and that the changes she was therefore introducing were necessary in the interests of patients. The foundation of her case was so secure that it could not reasonably be challenged. She appeared to have achieved the change without making the unqualified staff (whose role was substantially changed) feel devalued.

Pyne (1992a) points out how effective it would be if all practitioners who felt concern about standards communicated this in writing to their senior management. He points to the Access to Health Records Act 1991 and raises the point that if practitioners made honest and contemporaneous entries in patient and client records on situations in which care was compromised or could not be provided, this would have the effect of highlighting shortfalls and helping to ensure patient safety. As he says, 'Some managers will still choose to shoot the solitary messenger, rather than pay heed to the possibly accurate message'.

Dimond (1990) points out that it is clearly wrong for practitioners to pretend to be coping with the workload, to delude themselves into the conviction that things are better than they really are, to aid and abet the abuse and breakdown of a colleague or to tolerate in silence any matters in the work setting that place patients at risk, jeopardise standards of practice or deny patients' privacy and dignity. She also goes on to point out that the Code of Professional Conduct applies to all persons on the Council's register, irrespective of the post held and that while their perspective may vary with their role, they share the overall responsibility for care.

It is little understood that managers can be held accountable for the service that they offer and it is frequently the nurse on the lower rungs of the ladder who picks up the responsibility and who experiences problems in not having the resources, the facilities or the time to carry out the care adequately. In addition, the diminution of nursing management means that in certain situations nurses are reporting to non-nursing managers who, while being accountable to their employers, will not be accountable in the professional way that nurses are. There is a growing concern that some of these managers are not fully cognisant of the complexities and contexts of care.

The case of Beverly Allitt, the nurse who murdered four children, pointed up some of these problems. According to a report in *The Guardian* (1993) nurses and doctors at the Grantham and Kesteven Hospital repeatedly warned management that staffing levels on the paediatric ward were dangerously low. The nursing manager for the children's and maternity wards wrote to her boss requesting authorisation to hire more staff because she did not have enough nurses to cover for those who were ill or on holiday. No action was taken. She further wrote to say that the shortage of nurses with paediatric training on ward 4 meant that it had become an unsafe environment for children. The ward's night sister had written to consultants and hospital general managers stressing that night staffing on the ward was insufficient and that the ward's resuscitation equipment was inadequate and she requested that 'a solution be implemented before a tragedy occurs'. Tragically she herself committed suicide in September 1991 after Beverly Allitt was arrested. Other senior nurses warned that ward 4 did not have enough nurses to 'maintain a safe environment for the children in our care'. One senior nurse, Mary Reet, wrote, 'While I am fully aware of the present economic climate I do not feel I am justified in remaining silent about my concern'. In this particular case, there was a lack of managerial accountability and these warnings were ignored with very tragic consequences. It is important to note that there is a Department of Health circular on qualifications on paediatric wards and that the health authority had a policy for the staffing on paediatric wards.

Conclusion

Nurses, midwives and health visitors should be in no doubt about their responsibility to be accountable for their own practice in the interests of patient care. The changes in the health service make it imperative that they are informed and articulate about such responsibilities. The UKCC must take a more proactive role in speaking out on behalf of nurses and patients and make its position clear as soon as possible when issues arise in the media or in service. Nurses must feel their statutory body is behind them in offering the support necessary. Equally, nurses must not be afraid to use the Code of Professional Conduct to maintain standards.

References

DIMOND, B. (1989) Accountability in a legal context *Nursing Standard* **3(49)**, 29–31.

DIMOND, B. (1990) *Legal Aspects of Nursing*. Prentice Hall, Herts.

THE GUARDIAN (1993) Report on Beverly Allitt. 19/5/93, p. 4.

HEALTH VISITOR (1993) Report of MSF Survey **66(4)**, 115.

PYNE, R. (1992a) Breaking the code. *Nursing* **5(3)**, 8–10.

PYNE, R. (1992b) *Professional Discipline in Nursing, Midwifery and Health Visiting*. Blackwell, Oxford.

THOMPSON, I., MELIA, K. AND BOYD, K. (1988) *Nursing Ethics*. Churchill Livingstone, Edinburgh.

UKCC (1989) *Exercising Accountability*. UKCC, London.

UKCC (1992a) *Code of Professional Conduct*. UKCC, London.

UKCC (1992b) Registrar's letter of 14th December (ref 37/1992), Standards for Incorporation into Contracts for Hospital and Community Health Care Services. UKCC, London.

5

Community representation

Toby Harris

The UK health service has never been very open to external scrutiny. Similarly, the formal structures of its governance have never been particularly accountable to the public who use it. Many of the professions within the NHS are introverted and secretive. Moreover, the changes introduced by the NHS and Community Care Act 1990 have reduced accountability further and, if anything, made decision making even less transparent than it was before.

This chapter will look briefly at the 1991 changes and at the experience so far with the new NHS. It will also look at the history of community representation within the NHS and, in particular, at the role of community health councils.

The governance of the NHS before 1991

It has become something of a truism to say that the NHS has suffered a major reorganisation on average every three to five years since its creation in 1948. The details of its structure have changed many times. However, lines of accountability have tended throughout to go upwards towards government ministers rather than downwards towards the patients who use the service or towards the local community. This top-down approach has its origins in the formation of the service and the dictum of Aneurin Bevan that the sound of a dropped bedpan should resound down the corridors of Whitehall.

By the late 1980s, the structure of the NHS in England consisted of 14 regional health authorities (RHAs) whose members were appointed by the Secretary of State for Health. Each region was divided into districts and district health authorities (DHAs) had the responsibility for managing and planning most non-family practitioner services. The DHA chair was appointed by the Secretary of State and the vast majority of other members were appointed by the RHA (that is, appointed by nominees of the Secretary of State). A handful of DHA members were not so appointed: these were the local authority nominees. They rarely comprised more than a fifth of the total membership and were the only members who were able to claim any form of democratic legitimacy, albeit indirect.

In addition to the DHA and RHA structure was the organisation of the family practitioner services. Family doctors, dentists, pharmacists and opticians were not (and indeed, are still not) salaried NHS employees. Instead, they were independent contractors who had a contract with what was then called the family practitioner committee (FPC) to provide services to the local population. FPCs typically covered the area of several DHAs and (like RHAs) all of their members were appointed by the Secretary of State for Health and they were directly accountable to him.

DHAs were typically bodies of 16–19 members. FPCs were rather larger with 30 members. However, the dominance of government nominees in both types of body was assured. Although some of the members, particularly those on DHAs who were appointed by local councils, occasionally kicked over the traces, most of the time the government's line prevailed.

The inevitability of this was reinforced by the managerial chain of command. Unit general managers reported to district general managers, who in turn reported to regional general managers and they took the lead given by the chief executive of the NHS Management Executive. In cases where these managerial lines were insufficient, there was the mechanism of performance related pay, which meant that annual pay increases depended on the extent to which those in this chain of command convinced those one and two tiers above them of their achievement against objectives laid down from on high.

Thus it was perfectly possible for the Secretary of State to exercise a fairly tight control over the NHS. Guidelines issued by the Department were converted into objectives set for individual authorities and translated into performance targets for managers within those authorities. This process would be implemented both via the managerial structure and by pressure from health authority members who owed their appointment to the political patronage of government ministers.

Clear lines of accountability therefore existed in the health service before the changes brought about by the 1990 NHS and Community Care Act. However, the accountability was all upwards from local units via DHAs and RHAs to the Secretary of State. As far as the public was concerned, accountability was limited to the meetings of the DHAs, RHAs and FPCs and the existence of a small number of local council nominees on DHAs who had at least come through the electoral process. These meetings were by and large held in public but health bodies were covered by the Public Bodies (Admission to Meetings) Act 1960. This meant that they could resolve to go into private session whenever in their view publicity would be prejudicial to the public interest. In practice, this tended to be whenever controversial and difficult decisions were on the agenda.

In the mid-1980s a number of pieces of legislation were passed by Parliament, having been introduced as private members' bills, that sought to improve the public's access to decision making by public bodies. Thus, the Local Government (Access to Information) Act was passed in 1985. This specified and limited the circumstances in which local council meetings could be closed to the public and required that relevant documents (subject to certain exemptions) should be made available to members of the public on request. Subsequently, separate bills extended similar provisions to joint consultative committees (the bodies established to provide consultative arrangements between health authorities and local councils) and then to community health councils (CHCs – the local statutory patients' watchdogs). However, efforts to apply similar rules to DHAs and FPCs were not successful.

From the public point of view, therefore, the governance of the health service tended to be secretive and the structures were obscure. People did not understand the distinction in roles between the different health bodies and found the relationship between their family doctors (as independent contractors) and the NHS difficult to fathom. As can be seen below, the changes that followed the 1990 Act, if anything, made the structures even more opaque as far as the public were concerned and blurred accountability even more.

The changes following the NHS and Community Care Act 1990

The most significant element of the changes and reorganisation within the NHS that followed the 1990 Act and which came into effect from 1 April 1991 was the introduction of the internal market and the creation of the purchaser–provider split. The role of district health authorities was altered so that their core function became to purchase services on behalf of their local population. They were to purchase services from provider units, which could be NHS trusts, directly managed units or units in the independent sector. As directly managed units became trusts in successive waves in the years following the Act, DHAs ceased to have any responsibility for the direct provision of services.

DHAs were not, however, the only purchasers. General practitioners could opt, under certain circumstances, to become fundholders and act as purchasers for their patients. This meant that, unlike other GPs, they were not restricted in how they referred their patients. Their only constraint was the money in their budget. GPs who were not fundholders, however, were in practice expected to refer their patients to those units where their local DHA had placed a contract (unless they were prepared to seek approval on an individual basis for an 'extracontractual referral'). Another change was in the health authorities themselves. DHAs, RHAs and family health services authorities (the new bodies that effectively replaced FPCs) all became much smaller. Typically, a DHA might now have a chair, appointed by the Secretary of State, five executive members and five non-executive members. The executive members would include the senior fulltime employees of the authority and the non-executive members would have been appointed by the RHA. All the members would therefore be upwardly accountable, either by virtue of employment or by appointment. There was no longer a provision for those nominated by local authorities to have a place on health authorities. Trust boards are similar in structure with a mix of executive and non-executive members, again with no opportunity for local authority representation. Neither in health authorities nor in trusts is there any requirement that non-executive members should have links with the communities that they serve.

The role of the non-executive members of health authorities was changed significantly by the new structure. Instead of having a supervisory responsibility for the authority's activities, which included the work of the most senior employees, non-executive members now had equal status with executive members on the authority itself. If any of the non-executive members was absent from a meeting, they could now be outvoted by the executive members. Moreover, the tendency for the officers to dominate the discussions and decisions was now much stronger. In addition, the fact that the chief executive would be the line manager of the other executive members could give them an effective block vote of almost half the authority, if they chose to exercise power and influence in that way. In effect, the non-executive members could be easily sidelined in the new structure.

In any event, the meetings of Health Authorities appear to be of even less significance than they were prior to 1991. Certainly, the meetings are less frequent. Prior to the NHS reforms, virtually all DHAs held formal meetings 10–12 times a year. Now it would appear that only a quarter of DHAs do so, with 62% meeting only four–six times a year. The impression of CHCs has been that an increasing number of decisions are made outside these formal meetings and therefore away from public view (ACHCEW, 1993).

It may be argued, of course, that there is now less for DHAs to do. Purchasing is a less intensive activity, some would say, than managing and providing services. Nevertheless, there is clearly a trend towards less frequent meetings with many purchasing decisions being taken in private because of considerations of 'commercial confidentiality'. Given the changes in structure, DHAs as purchasers are certainly less accountable than their predecessors.

It cannot, however, be said that trusts, as the main providers in the new structure, in any way redress this balance. The split of membership of trust boards between executive and non-executive members mirrors that of health authorities. Given also that trusts are usually in competition with other service providers, the arguments about commercial confidentiality provide a powerful incentive for secretive and non-accountable decision making.

The statutory requirement is that trusts should hold one meeting a year that is open to the public. In practice, of course, most trusts hold formal meetings more often than that. CHCs report that 40% of trusts meet 10–12 times a year, 36% meet four–six times a year and 18% three times a year or less (ACHCEW, 1993). Many of these meetings will not be open to the public and a significant minority of trusts do no more than the bare minimum required by law and use that one occasion as a public relations opportunity.

For the public, the new structural arrangements seem even more remote and confusing than the previous arrangements. The concept of the purchaser–provider split is an opaque one to most service users. It is difficult to determine responsibility for decisions. For an individual, the failure to refer him or her to a particular facility may be a decision of the GP or it may be because the DHA no longer has a contract with that provider or has fully utilised its quota of referrals earlier in the financial year. The decision to stop providing a service at a particular location may be the consequence of an operational decision by the provider concerned or it may follow from the failure to win contracts or extracontractual referrals to the volume originally anticipated. Moreover, the contractual decision may have been taken not by one purchaser but by a whole series of purchasers all making small adjustments to their purchasing plans. Accountability becomes blurred under such circumstances.

The situation is made worse by the multiplicity of purchasing arrangements. An increasing proportion of the population now have their health services purchased by GP fundholders. GP fundholders are not accountable for their purchasing decisions to their patients or to the public at large, although they may be required to explain their purchasing arrangements to the RHA or, where delegated, to the FHSA. In addition, some fundholders have banded together into purchasing consortia, whose decisions are accountable only to the fundholders who comprise them.

At the same time many DHAs have merged into larger units, thereby becoming even more remote from the communities on whose behalf they are supposed to be buying services. Where these mergers have been formalised, then the comments made earlier about the operation of DHAs apply. However, in a number of cases DHAs work together (and sometimes with the FHSA) as part of a consortium or joint commissioning agency. There is even less obligation on such informal groupings than there is on DHAs to operate openly or in an accountable fashion.

The rhetoric surrounding the NHS and Community Care Act was about strengthening decision making and accountability. Thus, the government's 1989 White Paper promised that the changes would 'make the health service more responsive to the needs of patients' with 'as much power and responsibility as possible . . . delegated to local level' (DOH, 1989). The reality, however, has been that decision making within the NHS has become even more shrouded in mystery than before and that far from improving local accountability, it has been worsened and those taking decisions have become more remote and less accessible than ever before.

The role of community health councils

Nearly 20 years before the 1991 NHS reorganisation, concerns about the lack of democratic accountability and remoteness from the service user were already prevalent. Thus, as a byproduct of the 1973 reorganisation, community health councils were created as the 'patients' watchdog'. Christine Hogg suggests that there were a variety of reasons for creating CHCs (Hogg, 1986). Firstly, it was considered that a good model would be to separate management from the representation of patient and community interests. This followed scandals about care in some long-stay hospitals where it was felt that hospital management committees had had a conflict of interest in managing the service and seeking to protect patients' interests. Second, consumerism was a rising force. Third, CHCs would ensure that voluntary groups and lay interests would be represented in the NHS. Fourth, CHCs would provide for more local authority input into the NHS, something which was then considered important.

As was so often the case subsequently, the whole idea of CHCs seems to have been something of an afterthought with one minister quoted as saying, 'We first decided that there should be such a body and then decided what it should do. As we worked on the CHCs, we found more things for them to do' (Klein and Lewis, 1976).

In the event the NHS Reorganisation Act 1973 set up a CHC in each NHS district and laid the general duty on each CHC 'to represent the interests in the health service of the public in its district'. This is, of course, an extremely broad remit and the intention that the remit should be broad is evidenced by the statements made in the subsequent guidance (DHSS, 1974) which said that CHCs might wish to direct their attention to 'the effectiveness of services being provided in the health district and their adequacy in relation to health care needs . . . the planning of services . . . changes in services . . . standards . . .'. This in practice meant that no area of the NHS was excluded from the terms of reference of CHCs.

Given this wide remit and the fact that most CHCs were comparatively under-resourced, it is not surprising that individual CHCs have developed in a variety of ways and have interpreted this remit differently according to local circumstances. Typically, however, a CHC's work might be described as falling into two main areas. First, CHCs monitor the NHS in their local area and seek improvements in the way in which it operates. Typically, this might involve carrying out surveys to find out what local people need from the NHS, collecting information about local services and visiting hospitals, clinics and other NHS premises to assess the standards of care. It would also involve representing local interests when changes are proposed for local health services and making proposals for improvements in services. The second main area of work is providing help and advice to members of the public, in particular in advising and supporting individuals with complaints about the way in which they have been treated by the NHS.

The significance of CHCs is that they form a link between those who administer the NHS and the people who use it. Each CHC has between 18 and 24 members, made up of people from the local community. Half of the members are appointed by the local councils for the area. A third are elected by local voluntary groups and organisations and the remainder are appointed by the RHA. In addition, the CHC can co-opt people with specialist skills or a particular interest. CHC members are lay people who give their time voluntarily to seek improvements in local health care. Frequently they will, as individuals, be involved in a wide range of local groups and the CHC itself will maintain a network of organisations and community based groups with whom it keeps in regular touch. Often CHCs will arrange and facilitate meetings of service users, bringing them together with each other, the CHC members and those within the NHS who are responsible for the service they use. A particular focus in this is frequently to make sure that those groups who are usually from more formal consultation processes have the opportunity to put their points of view.

Crucial to all of this is the independence of CHCs from either the government or the local health authority structure. CHCs are the only bodies in the health service that elect their own chairs. The members are serviced and supported by a small secretariat, usually of two people, who are separate from the local health service management. RHAs are notionally the employers of CHC staff and provide the money for CHC budgets. Despite this, the independence of CHCs from the services they are monitoring locally has usually been protected. However, there is some evidence that RHAs are increasingly seeking to influence the way in which CHCs work in some parts of the country.

Hogg records that in their first few years CHCs were seen as an interesting and successful experiment and received favourable mentions in several government reports (Hogg, 1986). In 1979, the Royal

Commission on the NHS concluded that CHCs had 'made an important contribution towards ensuring that local public opinion is represented to health service management' (HMSO, 1979).

However, this contribution did not make CHCs universally popular. Some health service managers found it threatening and time consuming to have to respond to the views of CHCs and service users, and the post-1979 government found that CHCs tended to be hostile to its policies. Within months of the Royal Commission's report being published a government White Paper entitled, ironically, *Patients First* suggested that CHCs might be abolished, saying:

> The need for separate consumer representation . . . is less clear; next year the councils will cost over £4 million. The government will welcome views on whether community health councils should be retained when the new district health authority structure has been implemented.
>
> (DHSS, 1979)

In the event, as Hogg describes, there was wide opposition to the abolition of CHCs and they were given a reprieve, subject to a review in due course (Hogg, 1986). In practice, the future of CHCs remained uncertain throughout the 1980s and it was never clear whether the consumerist thorn in the flesh would be allowed to remain.

The major changes in the NHS contained in the NHS and Community Care Act were not intended to alter the remit and work of CHCs. Indeed, government ministers went on record as saying that there would be no change in their fundamental role. Two significant changes did, however, occur as a byproduct of the Act. The first related to consultation procedures. In the past one of the key rights of CHCs had been their right to be consulted by health authorities on any proposals for a major closure, a substantial development or variation of services. Inevitably, the introduction of the internal market and the purchaser–provider split has changed the nature of those items which come forward for formal consultation. The closure of a facility is now more likely to be the consequence of earlier contractual and purchasing decisions and as a result, consultation when the closure itself is proposed is too late for any influence to be meaningfully exerted. Consultation still takes place but it is carried out by the DHA rather than by the provider unit concerned. As a result, the limited accountability that previously existed through the requirement to consult publicly with the CHC has effectively been negated. While DHAs are still expected to consult about their purchasing plans, the process is often a rather nebulous one. Moreover, the purchasing decisions of GP fundholders may be critical in determining the future of any units and 90% of CHCS report that they have never been consulted about GP fundholders' purchasing plans (ACHCEW, 1993).

The second significant change affecting CHCs was the downgrading of CHCs' rights to observer status at health authority meetings. Prior to the 1990 Act ministerial guidance laid down that:

> The Secretary of State expects that the CHC should send one of its members to meetings of the matching DHA as an observer. These observers will have the same right as members of the authority to speak during meetings but will not vote. Observers will not automatically be excluded from those parts of the DHA meetings or committee meetings which are not open to the public . . . CHC observers should receive all papers to be discussed by DHAs.
>
> (DHSS, 1981)

Prior to the 1990 changes, all CHCs were invited to DHA meetings, 98% had speaking rights and only 11% were not allowed to stay for the private parts of meetings. This gave the public, through the CHC representative, an opportunity both to know what decisions were being taken by health authorities and to influence those decisions.

However, these opportunities were not a statutory right and were not enshrined in legislation and at the end of 1990 new guidance was issued. This replaced the earlier 'expectation' of the Secretary of State with the following formulation:

> CHCs have rights, as do other members of the public, to attend any NHS authority or NHS trust meeting open to the public. It is a matter for decision by NHS authorities and NHS trusts whether CHCs will be invited to address meetings which are open to the public or to attend meetings which otherwise are closed to the public.
>
> (NHS Management Executive, 1990)

This had the immediate effect of reducing the number of CHCs who were allowed to speak at authority meetings from 98% to 87% and 28% of CHCs were now not allowed to stay for the private parts of meetings. The figures for FHSAs were even worse, with only 80% allowed to speak and 67% of CHC representatives never allowed to stay for private sessions (ACHCEW, 1993). Although the figures have improved slightly since then, the accountability of the NHS to the public through CHCs took a severe knock as a result of these changes. What is more, the CHC involvement remains at the discretion of individual authorities: it can be withdrawn at any time and is presumably more likely to be withdrawn if the messages being delivered by the CHC representative are unpalatable.

Charterism and *Local Voices*

The overall effect, then, of the 1990 Act was to blur and diminish the accountability of the health service to the public. At the same time, community health councils, as the remaining mechanism whereby the views of the public could have formal access to the governance of the NHS, had had their ability to influence events restricted. Then towards the end of 1991 and early in 1992 a different approach to the NHS began to emerge. It coincided with the new 'softer' image being projected by the government, which cynics ascribed to the imminence of a general election.

Thus, in July 1991 'The Citizen's Charter' was launched. This pointed out that:

> In the past, the inspectors of our public services have usually been members of the profession they oversee. This has made for too close a relationship. The government wants to give people from different backgrounds a bigger say in the future.
>
> (HMSO, 1991)

The tone of the document was consumerist and the aim was alleged to make the public services more accountable to their users. The Citizen's Charter was followed a few months later by the publication of the Patient's Charter. This laid great emphasis on the NHS being a service that 'always puts the patient first, providing services that meet clearly defined national and local standards, in ways responsive to people's views and needs' and went on to stress the need for better information to the public and improving mechanisms for listening to the views of service users (DoH, 1991).

Whilst the two charters were in essence about service standards, they helped to create a climate in which those within the NHS began to think about how services could be made more responsive to the needs of patients. In January 1992 the NHS Management Executive issued *Local Voices* which considered how the views of local people might be fed into purchasing decisions (NHS Management Executive, 1992a). The following month, Stephen Dorrell MP, then the Parliamentary Under Secretary of State for Health, wrote to the chairs of health authorities encouraging them to facilitate the 'development of CHCs as the consumer representative in the purchasing function' (DoH, 1992) and this was followed up by a circular from Andrew Foster, Deputy Chief Executive of the NHS Management Executive, reiterating and spelling out this message to general managers and chief executives (NHS Management Executive, 1992b).

The key point in these documents was that the purchasing activities of health authorities must be rooted in the needs and wishes of local people, that a good working relationship between CHCs and health authorities is important in this and that CHCs should increase their focus on purchasing issues. The documents also recognised that CHCs should have reasonable access to the information on which health authorities base their judgements and also to the contracts of GP fundholders. They also accept that CHCs should have the opportunity to contribute to the process of local target setting, monitoring performance against the targets set, setting quality standards, monitoring performance against standards and assessing relative service priorities. Finally, it was made clear that health authorities should recognise the role given by Parliament to CHCs and ensure that the opportunity exists for them to fulfil this role (including adequate resourcing).

All of these developments indicated a much more positive approach to the idea of service user involvement in the new NHS and towards the role of CHCs than had been apparent at the time of the 1990 Act. However, the question remains as to how significant this more positive approach will be. *Local Voices* (NHS Management Executive, 1992a) cites a wide range of ways of obtaining the views of patients. The process nonetheless has a long way to go. Finding out the needs of service users is more than just carrying out the odd satisfaction survey. It needs to be a continuous process and one that has the commitment of the entire organisation. Considerable vigilance needs to be exercised to ensure that the *Local Voices* approach does not lead to what might be termed 'managed consumerism'.

Managed consumerism means maintaining the show of involving the users of service whilst at the same time making sure that it does not impede what those running the service intend to do in any case. This may mean 'consulting' when a decision is already finalised. It may mean getting the response that you want by the careful manipulation of the information provided to the users or handpicking the so-called representative users that are asked.

Initiatives by managers on setting up consultation mechanisms or even on reviewing the quality of service need to be independently validated. It is too easy to construct a survey's methodology so that it produces the answer required. Similarly, the questions put to focus groups or to consumer panels may be trivial or can simply be those to which the manager knows the answer. It is far too common, in any event, for a management led approach to omit the key issues as far as service users are concerned. If 'local voices' are genuinely to be heard and consultation exercises are to be real processes rather than simply going through the motions, service users need their own representative mechanisms, such as CHCs, which are independent of health authority structures. This would provide support and focus for the users and external, independent validation of the initiatives being taken by purchasers and providers to assess local views.

Conclusion

Patient empowerment creates a partnership between the patient and the service. Such a partnership will be essential for the future development of the NHS because it would help improve patient–staff relations, would help rebuild public confidence in a beleaguered NHS and thereby help boost morale in the service itself. Slow faltering steps are being taken by the NHS in the right direction to achieve this. That is why the efforts towards strengthening patients' rights, enhancing the voice of service users in decision making and promoting patient empowerment are so important.

Further progress will, however, require major cultural and institutional changes within the health service. First, genuine empowerment requires that those being empowered must be informed. Information phone lines and help desks may be helpful in this, but are often little more than gimmicks. Instead, what is required is that at every stage in a service user's encounter with the NHS all staff (whether medical, nursing or administrative) should share information with the service user on all aspects for their condition and care. It should be given readily and should be reinforced by well-produced background material appropriate to the user's needs. Service users should also have ready access to external information sources, but such a service must be independent of the service providers.

Second, when things go wrong, service users should have ready access to independent advice and support and there should be a user-friendly complaints system for them to pursue their concerns. The existing arrangements for investigating patient's complaints are bureaucratic, cumbersome, longwinded and strongly biased in favour of the medical profession (ACHCEW, 1990; see also Ch. 3).

Third, patients need their own independent representative structure to promote their interests in an increasingly market and finance driven environment. Such a structure should be an enabling one that encourages service users to put forward their views and facilitates community groups to feed into the NHS.

In all of these areas, CHCs could have a big role to play. However, the future remains uncertain. Revised guidance on the role of CHCs is again being prepared within the NHS Management Executive. Some RHAs remain sceptical about the role of CHCs and have pushed through mergers of CHCs, so that in some cases CHCs are expected to cover populations well in excess of half a million people, thereby rendering the community representatives themselves remote from the communities they are supposed to support.

None of the recent changes in approach to CHCs and to consulting and involving the community has any new statutory backing. They are no more than guidance in a legal framework that is designed to frustrate public accountability. It is therefore much too early to say whether the moves towards patient empowerment and consumerism are anything other than window-dressing to disguise a system that retains all its previous features of secretiveness, remoteness and central control.

References

ACHCEW (1990) *National Health Service Complaints Procedure*. ACHCEW, London.

ACHCEW (1993) *Association of Community Health Councils for England and Wales Annual Report 1992/93*. ACHCEW, London.

DoH (1989) *Working for Patients*. HMSO, London.

DoH (1991) *The Patient's Charter*. HMSO, London.

DoH (1992) *Community Health Councils ML(92)1*. HMSO, London.

DHSS (1974) *Community Health Councils HRC(74)4*. DHSS, London.

DHSS (1979) *Patients First*. HMSO, London.

DHSS (1981) *The Membership of District Health Authorities HC(81)6*. DHSS, London.

HMSO (1979) *The Royal Commission on the National Health Service*. HMSO, London.

HMSO (1991) *The Citizen's Charter*. HMSO, London.

HOGG, C. (1986) *The Public and the NHS*. ACHCEW, London.

KLEIN, R. AND LEWIS, J. (1976) *The Politics of Consumer Representation*. Centre for Studies in Social Policy, London.

NHS MANAGEMENT EXECUTIVE (1990) *Consultation and Involving the Consumer*. DoH, London.

NHS MANAGEMENT EXECUTIVE (1992a) *Local Voices*. DoH, London.

NHS MANAGEMENT EXECUTIVE (1992b) *Community Health Councils EL(92)11*. DoH, London.

6

Explaining abuse and inadequate care

David Pilgrim

The publication of the report of the inquiry into events at Ashworth Special Hospital (DoH, 1992) highlights the pressing need to understand the psychology and culture of health care institutions in relation to their accountability. Ashworth, like Rampton and the other special hospitals, is an extreme example of a dysfunctional care organisation. Its purported organisational goal of care was subordinated to other goals such as security and the needs and wants of staff. The bravery of the whistleblowers and the cruelty of the staff they sought to expose invite a psychological study.

Why do people who are paid to be carers sometimes engage in neglectful or cruel acts? Why do many others, who are not neglectful or cruel, act with complicity? Why do professionals fail to blow the whistle on the malpractice and misconduct they witness? What factors generate 'whistleblowers'?

Martin's book *Hospitals in Trouble* (1985) not only summarises the scandals occurring during the 1960s and 1970s about patient neglect and staff brutality, it also begins to address some of the key questions which need to be pursued regarding accountability and secrecy, bad practice and how to rectify it. Martin notes that whistleblowers are often people who are new to a system and who have not yet 'invested' themselves in it very much. For this reason, student nurses are quite likely to blow the whistle while nurse managers are not. This implies that the very people we might expect to be expert, professional and trustworthy informants about abuses are often the very ones who cover up and engage in a rhetoric of justification. Thus an uncharted area of social psychology concerns those factors surrounding collusion in failing health care institutions. No doubt these include fear of damage to career prospects, of losing reputation and status and even of losing one's job.

Traditional social psychological studies of conformity might inform research and training in this area (Asch, 1956; Crutchfield, 1955). These experiments demonstrated that under peer group pressure people will make irrational judgements about how they perceive events around them. Other social psychological investigations have shown that

normally benign people will act cruelly under experimental conditions·
which confer upon them the power to direct, humiliate or inflict pain
(Milgram, 1963; Zimbardo, 1972). Conformity and obedience which
lead to collusion with cruel practices are seen as resulting from group
pressures. A more individualistic explanation may be derived from psy-
choanalytical theory, in which sadistic tendencies are explained within a
psychosexual developmental framework (Adorno et al, 1950; Fromm,
1977; Menzies, 1977). Whether explanations from group dynamics are
privileged over those from personality characteristics or vice versa
remains a contested area.

Organisation and isolation

There is of course a danger in seeking explanations about dysfunctional
systems in psychology. Martin mentions whistleblowers and the perpetrators of neglect and abuse but he cautions against the 'bad apple' theory. It is comforting, perhaps, when faced with the organisational crisis
created by unspeakable acts in health care systems, to believe that psychological accounts are wholly adequate. The research noted above,
about sadism and conformity, may well invite this type of reductionist
explanation. However, there remains a tension within social science
between this psychological emphasis and the organisational context as
sources of explanation.

   In the scandal hospitals which Martin reviews, there are certain recur-
ring organisational characteristics. In particular, the acts of brutality or
neglect occurred in the context of several layers of isolation. The most
immediate layer was that of ward isolation. This encourages a sort of
'fiefdom' mentality among those running the ward and a preoccupation
with staff power and autonomy. This danger is greater the bigger the
organisation. Very large institutions are often governed by blanket rules
which apply throughout but at the same time contain isolated sub-
systems which may become a law unto themselves. For instance
recently a student nursery nurse has been imprisoned for sexually abusing boys and girls in his workplace. A series of unchecked incidents
took place under tables, when he molested the children's genitals and
then subsequently bullied the children into silence. This happened with
trained staff working within a few yards of each incident. Commentators
were puzzled about how such abuse could go undetected under the noses
of colleagues. Similarly, a series of suspicious deaths in special hospitals
has occurred in the 'seclusion' rooms within wards but none of these
cases has (at the time of writing) led to charges of unlawful killing.

   With this type of example in mind, we must ask how we can organise
caring work in a way which ensures that there is sufficient ongoing

mutual surveillance to pre-empt wrongdoing and abuse without infringing reasonable expectations of privacy and benign intimacy.

A second layer of isolation is that of the institution itself. Many places in which problems have occurred have been geographically isolated. We need only think about the old institutions which 'warehoused' psychiatric patients and people with learning difficulties to understand the separation of these places from community scrutiny. Tall boundary walls and security moats keep their inmates in and the evaluative gaze of others out.

The brutality at Rampton was exposed by a television programme using accounts of ex-inmates (DHSS, 1980). When four years later, in the wake of the 1983 Mental Health Act, the Mental Health Act Commission was set up there were hopes that this would prevent a recurrence of such incidents. In 1991, after seven years of regular visits by commissioners to Ashworth Hospital, it took another media exposé to bring its problems to light. This failure of the Commission highlights how isolated institutions can be impermeable to external accountability. It also demonstrates that responsible journalism can sometimes achieve more in one act of reporting than the ongoing activity of official watchdogs.

A third layer of isolation is that of the health care practitioners. When health care scandals have occurred it is not uncommon to find that the staff involved had become isolated from their professional discipline. They then develop peculiar norms of daily practice which would perplex or shock colleagues from elsewhere. This poses a particular problem for the care professions. Apart from laying down codes of practice, how are standards actually enforced?

Graham Pink, the Stockport nurse who exposed inadequate care of the elderly on the wards of his hospital, thought that his code of practice and regulatory body would vindicate and support his actions, but he was disappointed. His case also highlights another sort of professional isolation: in hospitals, which might generally maintain good care standards in terms of practice norms and staffing levels and other resources, there is a pecking order of status within medical specialties. At the bottom of this order are patients who are often disvalued such as elderly people and those diagnosed as being mentally ill. Staff working with these people may become isolated from the norms of others working with other patients in the same hospital.

Prejudice and discrimination

Pink's case spurred a whole string of published and private correspondence from nurses working elsewhere with elderly patients, confirming a very similar picture of under-resourcing and consequent patient neglect. This was often contrasted with better staffing levels and resources on wards which were more 'heroic'. Professional and public concerns about standards may be contaminated by ageism and other prejudices. Is accountability enforced more for the benefit of some patients than others?

It is now well established that black and Irish people are over-represented in psychiatric inpatient populations, especially in secure provision, and that they are subjected to higher drug dosage regimes than white British patients (Pilgrim and Rogers, 1993). Why does this occur and why is it tolerated by so many inside and outside the caring professions? The answer must lie both in the racial disadvantage which affects the well-being of these black and ethnic minorities and the prejudicial way they are then treated by professionals. Where is this racist power held to account currently within care systems?

The client group as a predictor of poor care is addressed by Martin in terms of patients who are 'unrewarding' – those who are slow or impossible to habilitate or rehabilitate. This narrow framing of patient characteristics is obviously not wholly predictive of resourcing and care levels, in the light of what has just been mentioned about intensive care wards which have a very high mortality rate. Generally, though, Martin's point is a fair one, but it might be better understood in terms of the *value* that is placed on some patients but not others. Those younger patients who do recover from traumatic injury can be celebrated as the 'heroic' rescue of youth and health from the jaws of death and disability. This concurs with the image of medicine which professionals and lay people find comforting or exciting. By contrast, those who are old, have degenerative disabilities, mental health problems or learning difficulties may be unrewarding and they are coincidentally poorly valued by wider society. Professional attitudes will reflect such social attitudes. In turn these values are shaped in part by the question of the economic value of subgroups in the population – an issue I will return to below. Should the problem of accountability be addressed without exploring this question of some patients being valued less than others?

When there is a confluence or aggregation of these factors of isolation and prejudice then neglect and brutality are highly predictable. Since Martin's review of the scandal hospitals with these aggregating or 'synergistic' features, we have also witnessed similar organisational features in residential social work – the Staffordshire pin-down scandal and the series of exposés about paedophiles abusing young people in their care in North Wales and Leicester are cases in point. The versions of isolation and the low social value placed on disruptive young people came together to offer a setting in which power could be easily abused.

Organisational values

One of the striking features about this area in historical context is that there has been a discursive shift over the past 200 years about which values are implicit to health care policy. As far as chronic disabling conditions are concerned, the hospital has been the target of debates about segregation and desegregation. There has been the question as to whether hospitals should permanently house disvalued (or 'deviant') people. Until relatively recently the hospital has sustained a more conflict free image as being a legitimate site for the optimal application of scientific medicine to *acute* conditions.

For different reasons both forms of hospital use, chronic and acute, are now under critical scrutiny. The recent Tomlinson Report about teaching hospitals in London highlights an emerging concern about prioritising secondary sector goals over those of community based health care facilities. Likewise, the rise of the hospice movement has increasingly challenged the organisation of death within the rules of hospital based medicine, rather than on the basis of the expressed needs of dying people (Glaser and Strauss, 1965, 1968). Thus the social organisation of care has shifted with social values about life, death and suffering.

A dramatic example is the systematic killing of mentally and physically disabled patients by some German doctors during the Second World War (Meyer, 1988; Procter, 1989). The Nazis had a particular enthusiasm for a set of eugenic ideas that actually pervaded Western Europe and the United States at the end of the nineteenth and beginning of the twentieth centuries. The pseudoscience of eugenics warned of the dangers from foreign and lower class stock enfeebling the general population. Sickness and disability were understood within this framework as resulting from a 'tainted gene' pool which also produced other forms of deviance such as aggressive and criminal behaviour. The aim was the removal of all these manifestations of deviance from society (in the workhouse, the epileptic colony, the lunatic asylum, the prison and the infirmary) and the separation of sexes rigorously applied. Sterilisation of these patients was still common during the 1930s in Denmark and the United States, showing that eugenic ideas pervaded beyond and preceded Nazi Germany.

Accountability implies that health care goals are being met and are seen to be met. Within the eugenic euthanasia framework, before and during the Second World War, killings and the systematic denial of both the liberty and sexual freedom of patients were explicit health care goals. They were 'good' practice according to the professional norms of the times. So when we talk about accountability we need to recognise that these norms shift over time and place.

This helps us highlight two distinct types of whistleblowing. The first is where a professional draws attention to the conduct of colleagues which *violates* norms. An example here would be the 'Ashworth Four' who spilled the beans on bad practice in a secure psychiatric hospital. The second is where a professional *challenges* the norm itself, and thereby raises the question of whether it should be changed. An example here is the Pink case. His managers did not fundamentally dispute many of his factual claims about staffing levels. What they disagreed with was whether those were reasonable and appropriate levels. As the subsequent correspondence with Pink shows he was only really putting on record events he found unacceptable but that were commonplace elsewhere and even judged by many to be unremarkable.

Thirty years ago tonsillectomies were common practice. Now they are neither common nor usually legitimate. Antibiotics were prescribed in a cavalier way; now they are given out with caution. Will the current fashion for the surgical treatment of 'glue ear' go the same way in another 30 years? There is a need to explore two distinct questions about good and bad practice which draw attention to the question of norms. First, how is bad practice eliminated or reduced in health care systems (and good practice encouraged)? Second, how can we critically appraise whether current conceptions of good practice are fair and reasonable?

These questions are highly contested in sociology. Since the 1970s, the emphasis has been on the social construction of disability and illness (Armstrong, 1983; Oliver, 1990). This has made older, more certain definitions about what constitutes sickness and disability problematic, because the phenomena are seen as socially relative. Relativism ensures sensitivity about different times and places. But as recent critics point out (Doyal and Gough, 1991), it can take us to a position in which we can never say anything with any certainty about what a health care need is. What is certain, though, is that we cannot explore accountability about standards in health care unless we struggle with defining what needs are and who should *control* such definitions.

Currently a three-cornered fight seems to be occurring about need definition between service managers, service users and clinical professionals. Sometimes they concur and sometimes they do not. The new consumerism of the 1980s and the principles of industrial management in the NHS have stimulated this three-cornered battle, as has the emergence of the new social movement of disaffected health care users (Doyal, 1983; Oliver, 1990; Rogers and Pilgrim, 1991). Prior to these times, needs were defined by medical practitioners more or less without challenge.

User movements lie outside traditional parliamentary and local democratic structures and outside the traditional conflict between employers and workers. Indeed, in the case of health they are often organised by physically and mentally disabled people, who are largely outside the labour market, and by women, who have had less status and power within that market (Doyal, 1983).

Whilst there has been an emphasis within health policy over the past 10 years to encourage consumerism, the outcome for these groups is by no means clear at present. With marketisation and the purchaser–provider split the trend has been to place power in the hands of *purchasers* of services (health authorities). These may exercise discretion over how they involve service users. It may only be limited to satisfaction surveys of individual consumers as a quality control check and may not involve giving collective power to service users in planning and delivering services (see Ch. 5).

Resources

Those opposed to marketisation and cash limits in the NHS have repeatedly drawn attention to resources. Do resources guarantee good practice and can the failures of health care services be understood ultimately in terms of how much is spent on those services? Is the most important condition of health care accountability our commitment to financial investment? Critics from health care systems from both left and right have tended to agree that such systems can consume increasing budgets without improvements in quantity or quality.

Explanations which are financially reductionist in this way would exclude from our consideration all of the other contextual features noted above, which feed into both good and bad practice. The contrast between the Ashworth scandal and Graham Pink's complaints shows how finance can be either all-important or irrelevant depending on the context. The special hospitals were (and remain) highly resourced and yet they have failed as health care institutions. However, in the case of understaffing of care of the elderly wards, more money would have probably made the difference between Pink being sacked for his whistleblowing and serving out his nursing days in quiet anonymity.

What these cases draw attention to is a wider question about linking finance to goals, which brings us back to the social organisation of values. For instance, we know that morbidity and mortality are linked to social class and that antipoverty measures would reduce this class gradient. A reduction in economic inequality in society would lead to a reduction in health inequalities (Doyal, 1979; Doyal and Gough, 1991). In fact what we have seen, by and large, since the Second World War is Western governments allowing such inequalities to be moulded by the vagaries of the national and international economy. At the same time they have exercised control over health care budgets as a proportion of gross national product. Health policy has largely meant the financing of *illness services*, not the pursuit of a wider social and economic policy to promote health equality.

Conclusion

Critics of rhetorical defences of inefficient or mystifying organisations have made the point that purported goals may not be achieved because they were never meant to be achieved (Etzioni, 1961). Also, as Baker (1971) notes: 'It is easy to confuse the convenient public fictions of official pronouncements with the actual functioning of a system'. This whole question of the relationship between rhetoric, unstated organisational goals and the political economy of health has taken on an intense quality over the past 10 years. If there is any doubt that hidden organisational goals are in operation and are disguised by managerial rhetoric, it is worth reflecting on the Pink and Ashworth/Rampton cases again. In the former, a nurse who acted with complete integrity, and in accord with both professional ethics and everyday decency, was dismissed by his managers for challenging their rhetoric about care standards. In the case of the special hospitals, nurses who assaulted and neglected patients retained their employment. This paradox points clearly to the gap which Baker and Etzioni describe.

General management has brought with it the requirement for clinicians to be more accountable but it has also brought a new form of mystification about health care. 'Mission statements' and glossy literature are the echo of the market favoured by current government in Britain. Whereas doctors once warded off accountability through their arcane knowledge and their restrictive practices, managers now do the same by means of public relations. Whilst doctors professionalised healing and at the same time disguised the pursuit of self-interest and power, they did at least establish explicit criteria of good and bad practice. Managers presently have no such criteria (save the aims set by budgets). Consequently, they are prone to a sort of ethical anarchy. Because they are governed by the market place and are rewarded by performance related payments, selling their actual or purported achievements becomes an end in itself and brings with it the danger of the professionalisation of insincerity in health care.

References

ADORNO, T. W., FRENKEL-BRUNSWICK, E., LEVINSON, D. F. AND SANFORD, R. N. (1950) *The Authoritarian Personality*. Harper, New York.

ARMSTRONG, D. (1983) *Political Anatomy of the Body*. Cambridge University Press, Cambridge.

ASCH, S. E. (1956) Studies of independence and conformity. A minority of one against a unanimous majority. *Psychological Monographs* **70**, whole of number 416.

BAKER, F. (1971) The changing hospital organisational system. In *Man in Systems*, M. D. Rubin (ed.) Gordon and Breach, New York.

CRUTCHFIELD, R. S. (1955) Conformity and character. *American Psychologist* **10**, 191–8.

DoH (1992) *Report of the Committee of Inquiry into Complaints about Ashworth Hospital*. HMSO, London.

DHSS (1980) *Report of the Review of Rampton Hospital*. HMSO, London.

DOYAL, L. (1979) *The Political Economy of Health*. Pluto, London.

DOYAL, L. (1983) Women, health and the sexual division of labour: a case study of the women's health movement in Britain. *Critical Social Policy* **7**, 21–33.

DOYAL, L. AND GOUGH, I. (1991) *A Theory of Human Need*. MacMillan, London.

ETZIONI, A. (1961) *A Comparative Analysis of Complex Organisations*. Free Press, Glencoe, Ill.

FROMM, E. (1977) *The Anatomy of Human Destructiveness* Penguin, Harmondsworth.

GLASER, B. G. AND STRAUSS, A. L. (1965) *Awareness of Dying*. Aldine, Chicago.

GLASER, B. G. AND STRAUSS, A. L. (1968) *Time For Dying*. Aldine, Chicago.

MARTIN, J. P. (1985) *Hospitals in Trouble*. Blackwell, Oxford.

MENZIES, I. (1977) *The Functioning of Social Systems as a Defence Against Anxiety*. Tavistock Institute, London.

MEYER, J. E. (1988) The fate of the mentally ill in Germany during the Third Reich. *Psychological Medicine* **18**, 575–81.

MILGRAM, S. (1963) Behavioral study of obedience. *Journal of Abnormal and Social Psychology* **67**, 371–8.

OLIVER, M. (1990) *The Politics of Disablement*. Macmillan, London.

PILGRIM, D. AND ROGERS, A. (1993) *A Sociology of Mental Health and Illness*. Open University Press, Milton Keynes.

PROCTOR, R. (1989) *Racial Hygiene: Medicine Under the Nazis*. Harvard University Press, Cambridge, Mass.

ROGERS, A. AND PILGRIM, D. (1991) 'Pulling down churches': accounting for the British mental health users movement. *Sociology of Health and Illness* **13**(2), 129–48.

ZIMBARDO, P. (1972) Pathology of imprisonment. *Trans-Action* **9**, 4–8.

Part Two

The Workplace and the Law

7

Self-regulation through employee vigilance

Marlene Winfield

> Every NHS manager has a duty to ensure that staff are easily able to express their concerns through all levels of management to the employing authority or trust. Managers must ensure that any staff concerns are dealt with thoroughly and fairly.
>
> (DoH, 1993, 3(ii))

> This ceaseless – almost overwhelming at Ashworth in recent years – flow of unresolved complaints from patients and inmates provides ample proof that the pressures upon staff who have witnessed or become aware of ill-treatment of patients by working colleagues, or of poor living conditions in the hospital, reveals as intractable a problem as society can imagine.
>
> (HMSO, 1992)

In the chapters that follow contributors will look at legal aspects of whistleblowing and accountability and the need for legal reforms. Yet one of the most effective forms of self-regulation in health care must surely be the vigilance of individual workers. If this is acknowledged by everyone, including the Health Secretary, why is it so rarely put into practice? Indeed, in the light of the Ashworth Inquiry's findings and the stories told in the first chapter of this book, the Department of Health's free speech *Guidance* (DoH, 1993) might look like the triumph of hope over experience.

Noblesse oblige?

Will the culture of openness indicated in the NHS guidelines ever become a widespread reality? Will the whistleblower hotline become a thing of the past? The answers to both questions depend on whether certain barriers to open communication can be removed. Let us look at a few of them.

Hospitals are closed social systems, wrapped in cloaks of medical confidentiality. The people who work in them work hard. Their long and unsociable hours can limit their contacts with people outside the hospital environment, which can narrow perspectives. In the most extreme cases, their livelihoods, their friendships and their leisure activities can all revolve around the hospital, breeding a fierce loyalty to colleagues and to the institution.

In hospitals, there is usually a well-defined pecking order, which is maintained by and which also controls the decision making process. This power structure serves to maintain the status quo.

Traditionally, senior medical staff have been the 'aristocracy', organised in fiefdoms or firms, to whom all others deferred. And like any good aristocracy, it has tended to do things the way they have always been done. After all, most consultants did not get where they are today by rocking the boat. Junior doctors and medical students are the heirs in waiting, engaged in the delicate business of proving themselves fit for status and privilege, only likely to rock the boat when made foolhardy by exhaustion.

The hospital's 'middle class' is made up of nurses, administrative staff and non-medical professionals – psychologists, social workers, physiotherapists, etc. The latter may have a certain independence of mind born of not being complete insiders, but they usually lack a power base from which to exert influence. Nursing staff are the stalwarts of health care. Enabling the system, however creaky, to continue to function is what is expected of them by their profession, at times by their unions and certainly by the public. Martyrdom can become a perverse source of satisfaction in the absence of rewards such as money and power.

Ancillary staff – porters, cleaners, laboratory assistants, nursing auxiliaries, etc. – can be seen as the low paid and disaffected 'working classes', their efforts rarely recognised let alone rewarded, their opinions rarely sought or taken seriously.

In this scheme, patients can be regarded as the 'deserving (and at times undeserving) poor', expected to be grateful for what they get. Everyone else in the hospital has a duty to look after them but not to engage with them much beyond that.

Recent reforms have shaken up this power structure. Hospital managers, once part of the quiescent middle class, are now emerging as the thrusting 'nouveaux riches'. With their fingers firmly on the hospital pursestrings, they are increasingly in a position to challenge the authority of consultants, as the British Medical Association and others now regularly lament.

A letter which appeared in *The Guardian* in February 1993 seems to reflect the frustration of an aristocracy surrendering its power to arrivistes with different priorities. Under the title 'Dissent that dare not speak its name', Professor Harry Keen, Chair of the NHS Support Federation, refers to a letter published earlier which in 'moderate and measured terms' criticised recent NHS reforms. Professor Keen speculates why the earlier letter had not been signed by the doctor who wrote it:

> It is clearly his or her perception that identification might attract reprisal, an unhealthy view which is now widespread in my profession which used to pride itself on its freedom to speak out, any time, anywhere, in the patient's interest.
> A disinclination to upset an all-powerful management, to be labelled 'subversive' and to suffer the consequences in career advancement, income or reputation has spread like a virus through the NHS. The commercial fidelity enforced in the business world has been imported into this great public service where attention to competitive advantage has assumed a new and unwelcome prominence.

In an environment where decision making is not shared, opinions and values tend to polarize. In hospitals coming to terms with controlling their own budgets, priorities can seem to diverge dangerously. Where the consultant's first priority may be to treat all those who need treatment and the nurse's to ensure that each patient is cared for properly during treatment, the manager's first priority must be to enable the hospital to remain solvent so that it can go on treating patients in the future.

While all of these goals are admirable and complementary, they can begin to seem mutually exclusive when not discussed. Nurses may object to taking on all who need treatment because it makes it impossible for them to provide an acceptable standard of care with the resources at hand. Managers may encourage treatment of certain patients and discourage treatment of others because of funding arrangements with health authorities and GPs which affect cash flows and ultimately the resources available to nurses and doctors to do their work. Being asked to favour certain patients and turn away others on economic grounds may improve cash flows but cause ethical dilemmas for both doctors and nurses. Each group may have a very different view of what is a proper staff-to-patient ratio. In the absence of forums to hear differing opinions and hammer out compromises, discontent can be left to seethe below the surface, looking for outlets.

News management

At the same time, new funding arrangements which put hospitals in competition with one another make it vital for each competing hospital to appear to be running smoothly. As in commercial companies, competition places an increasing premium on maximising the good news and minimising the bad. In such a climate, those with concerns about patient care can come to be seen not as conscientious team members but as troublemakers. If these messengers persist in bringing top management bad news, and worse still, if they share their concerns with outsiders, then for the good of the hospital they must be 'shot' – as Professor Keen suggests and as consultant haematologist Helen Zeitlin, nurse Graham Pink and others can testify.

To recap what are broad but I think accurate generalisations: present day hospital culture is shaped in part by the need to preserve patient confidentiality, a fierce code of loyalty, a strong sense of duty, a hierarchical power structure geared to resisting change and new funding arrangements which put a premium on competition and marketing. These factors combine to foster a culture which denies all but a few the power to make decisions and discourages the many from trying to influence decision making. What in other cultures might be regarded as employee vigilance or professionalism then becomes dissent that must be neutralised.

Healthy corporate management styles

How can such a culture be made more open? And how can self-regulation through vigilance be incorporated into new funding and contracting arrangements in the NHS? As hospitals are increasingly being run along business lines, perhaps something can be learned from looking at best practice in commercial companies.

For a decade or more in the private business sector (and more recently in the NHS), management has been elevated to an art form. Innumerable books are available, sharing the secrets and theories of successful managers. Management training courses and management consultants abound. While management developments in the NHS still tend to concentrate on cost effectiveness, many commercial companies have moved on to other aspects of management. Phrases like 'corporate culture' and 'industrial democracy' are bandied about not only in companies with touchy-feely management styles like Marks and Spencer and Body Shop, but also in more macho companies like ICI and BP.

German and Japanese management styles, where lines between managers and employees blur, are slowly infiltrating British boardrooms. While few British companies have yet achieved effective collective decision making as a method of self-regulation, some are taking cautious steps in that direction.

Is there a model of this type of self-regulation that both companies and the NHS can aspire to? A survey I conducted into self-regulation and whistleblowing in 53 British companies may hold clues (Winfield, 1990).

Where are we going?

The first requirement for self-regulation through employee vigilance is a willingness for it to happen. In the best companies this will come from the very top of the management tree – from the chair and chief executive. A clear message will be sent to all employees that their involvement is sought and welcomed.

Company mission statements are fashionable these days. They encompass in a few sentences what the company is here to do. For example:

> Bulmer drinks is committed to maintaining its leadership in the cider market and to building upon its strength as a leading independent manufacturer and distributor of branded premium non-alcoholic and alcoholic drinks. . . .
>
> (H. P. Bulmer)

> We want to be recognised as the world's most consistently successful company in the businesses we know best – hotels, catering and related services. . . .
>
> (Trust House Forte)

> To deliver the 'best value' independent health financing and insurance. To provide an unrivalled service to our customers. To pursue excellence and superior performance. To care for customers, staff, our suppliers and the community within where we operate.
>
> (BUPA)

> NFC will seek to become a company for all seasons. It will achieve this by developing a broad-based international, transport, distribution, travel and property group with a high reputation for service in all its activities. . . .
>
> (National Freight Company)

Some mission statements are drafted by outside consultants, some by boards. In the most progressive companies, the whole workforce will be involved in determining the company's mission through competitions, representation on committees or open forums.

While it is easy to be cynical about mission statements, the process by which they are devised and agreed can be very constructive and also revealing. If done in a spirit of cooperation, it allows workers at all levels to meet together to discuss what they are doing and why. In hospitals, the process might also involve patients and their families.

How will we get there?

Mission statements, even those arrived at by consensus, are not in themselves sufficient. Once all have agreed the destination, ground rules need to be set for the journey: what are we prepared and not prepared to do in order to get there?

Basic priorities will need to be agreed. These are sometimes embodied in a code of ethics. For example:

> ...To guard the good reputation of the Force, to work constantly to maintain its high ideals, to encourage others to do so by good example and leadership, and to contribute to its excellence by showing resolution and honesty if faced with police malpractice.
>
> (Metropolitan Police)

> Overly ambitious employees might have the mistaken idea that we do not care how results are obtained as long as we get the results. They might think it best not to tell higher management all that they are doing, nor to record all transactions accurately in their books and records, and to deceive the Company's internal and external auditors. They would be wrong on all counts.
>
> (Esso)

> ... employees must avoid any situation which makes them appear to have accepted a favour from somebody outside the Company, in the context of their work. It is much wiser to refuse today than to risk one's reputation tomorrow. If in any doubt say no, or seek management's approval in writing.
>
> (Rolls Royce)

> Key questions which may help understanding of the ethical aspects of our dealings with customers and suppliers include: Do our actions or proposed actions fall comfortably within Group guidelines, the consensus view of what constitutes ethical behaviour and generally accepted concepts of fairness and honesty? Might our actions mislead or raise expectations which cannot be fulfilled?...
>
> (BP)

Like mission statements, codes of ethics are most effective when workers at all levels have been involved in agreeing the priorities they embody.

Once basic priorities are agreed, further guidance may be needed to translate them into operating principles. Companies sometimes do this in codes of practice. Nurses, doctors and other clinical staff will be bound by their own professional codes. In some cases, so will managers. Trying to turn various professional codes and private value systems into an agreed workplace code can be an extremely effective way of uniting the workforce, although the process can at times be painful. In a culture trying to become more open, it at least enables suppressed feelings and concerns to be aired in a constructive way rather than as grievances, complaints, leaks and whistleblowing.

Once codes have been agreed, employees will need to be given a clear duty to put them into practice. Again, it is far better that this duty be seen as quality enhancement than as policing. Ideally, upholding agreed standards will be deemed to be the first loyalty employees owe to the workplace and to each other. If agreed standards have taken sufficient account of professional codes, the two should rarely come into conflict. When they do, at least there is a firm basis for negotiation.

Taking passengers

Once a workplace agrees a mission and codes, they need to be seen to inform the corporate strategy, the decision making process and day-to-day operations at all levels. At first, conscious efforts may need to be made to relate standards to decisions both major and minor; later this will probably become more or less automatic.

In enterprises serious about self-regulation, codes and missions will be prominently displayed where employees and managers can see them and be constantly reminded. Customers, suppliers, shareholders – or patients and their families – will be told of their existence and the implications for themselves.

For agreed standards to continue to inform a culture, all new employees, from day one, will need to be made aware of the mission and codes and their duties regarding them. Care will need to be taken at induction to ensure that standards and priorities are understood by all and that the process by which they are agreed and maintained is also understood.

Everyone's on-the-job training, from the office junior's to the chair's, from the porter's to the chief executive's, needs to contain a review of workplace values and standards and how to put them into practice. This will apply equally to training for promotion and management.

Of course, organisations do not stand still. Goals and objectives change, new dilemmas arise for which new guidance is needed. Therefore, missions and codes and the standards they embody will need to be reviewed and amended fairly regularly, ideally by consensus.

Putting self-regulation to the test

What happens when an employee with a clear duty to uphold workplace standards becomes concerned about possible lapses? Any organisation which is serious about self-regulation will want to have channels through which employee concerns can be heard and acted on. The point of entry might be an individual or a committee.

In the most progressive companies, employees might be encouraged to bring their concerns to an interdisciplinary employee/management committee with a wide-ranging brief, a committee with a specific area of responsibility such as health and safety or one concerned solely with product or service enhancement such as a quality circle.

Some companies operate 'open door' policies, encouraging employees to bring the most serious concerns directly to senior managers, in some cases directly to the main board. Others have designated officers – sometimes called ethics officers, registrars or stress counsellors – to hear employee concerns and take them up with appropriate managers. Still others operate confidential complaints procedures where employee concerns are given in writing to a designated officer, who removes any identification, passes them on to the appropriate senior manager, receives the reply and passes it back to the employee. A few companies regularly survey the workforce to solicit concerns, which are then taken up by a designated officer.

Where there is a cooperative management style, a concern, once expressed by an individual, becomes a concern of the workplace. The committee or designated officer takes on the ownership of the concern and takes on the task of raising it at the appropriate level, pursuing it and then reporting back. This reduces the chance of any individual being exposed or marginalised, victimised or driven to blow the whistle outside.

The Department of Health's *Guidance* on freedom of speech for NHS staff proposes its own procedures for dealing with staff concerns. The Department suggests that staff concerns which cannot be resolved locally be taken up the line, if necessary all the way to the general manager or chief executive of the hospital and in the last resort to the chair of the authority or trust. There is also some suggestion in the *Guidance* that the brief of the Health Services Ombudsman might be extended to offer an independent, external assessment of selected staff concerns which internal procedures have failed to address.

The procedure as conceived by the Department of Health is in danger of placing too heavy a burden on the individual staff member. In a culture based on co-operative management, the concern of a staff member needs to become a workplace concern at a very early stage and certainly before it reaches the chief executive or chair of the authority. Workplace committees or designated officers need to take clear responsibility for acting on concerns or for taking them up the line and this needs to be spelled out in the guidelines.

Where concerns are about allocation of resources, as many at present appear to be, then the sensible approach might be to involve the immediate staff team in considering the problem and finding workable compromises. In terms of good management, this must surely be preferable to shooting the messenger and expecting the survivors to struggle on in a climate of decay and fear.

It cannot be said often enough that staff concerns about patient care ought not be channelled through grievance or complaints procedures. This point is made quite firmly in the Ashworth Inquiry Report. In recommending the setting up of an incident review committee of patient representatives plus representatives from nursing, psychiatry, psychology, social work and administration, the Report observes:

> ...the (Special Hospitals Service) Authority has failed to appreciate, as was repeatedly said by many parties at the seminar, that incident reporting is a distinct and separate function from a complaints system. We are quite clear in our minds that such a committee as we propose, with a constant overview of what is going on daily in the hospital, is crucial to hospital management's commendable and visionary aim to produce a cultural change at Ashworth.
>
> (HMSO, 1992)

Regular check-ups

In a culture where staff are encouraged to raise concerns, there are likely to be systems for monitoring how well the channels of communication are operating

Do staff feel able to share their concerns? Are they taken up in an appropriate way? Are they acted on? Is the staff member kept informed of any action, involved in finding remedies or at least given an explanation when no action is taken? Are the majority of those who raise concerns satisfied with the outcome? Is anyone penalised for raising a concern? Is anyone rewarded? Could procedures for dealing with concerns be improved?

A few companies have strategies for monitoring performance in this area. Some have yearly 'ethical audits', which may include questions about internal communication systems. Some conduct exit interviews with employees leaving the company. Others regularly survey the workforce, including in the survey an assessment of procedures for sharing concerns. Others combine assessment with periodic reviews of codes and standards. Any of these methods might be adapted for use in hospitals.

Self-regulation: first steps

How does one begin to transform the culture of the hospital portrayed at the beginning of this chapter to one where all staff work together to maintain the highest possible standards of care (perhaps a more positive way of describing self-regulation)? I would suggest four initial steps.

First, the *Department of Health needs to take a firm lead in encouraging self-regulation.* Its *Guidance* (DoH, 1993) needs to be a good deal clearer, more even-handed and less ambivalent. For example, in warning staff against breaching their duty of confidence, the first draft neglected to point out that breaches can sometimes be justified in law if they are deemed to be 'in the public interest'. Before the free speech initiative goes any further, the public interest defence to breach of confidence needs to be properly acknowledged by the Department of Health. Moreover, a shared ownership approach to concerns needs to be clearly promoted in the *Guidance.*

Second, *health authorities, professional bodies and unions need to come together to agree terms of employment contracts* so that conflicts between professional codes, workplace values and terms of employment are minimised. For example, the limits of confidentiality need to be agreed and spelled out. Rights and duties of employees to raise concerns about standards of care need to be agreed and any limits to them spelled out. As long as this continues not to happen, seemingly conflicting demands will drive conscientious workers to blow the whistle outside – a state of affairs which is far from ideal.

Third, expectations need to be changed. *Education and training of future health care workers and managers need to promote a consensus model of management.* Medical schools, nursing schools, health care management courses, etc. need jointly to review their curricula with a view to working together to break down 'class' barriers so that decision making is shared more widely. *Health service managers need to draw up a professional code of their own* which dovetails with the codes of other health care professionals.

Fourth, *staff and patients in hospitals need to begin trying out co-operative self-regulation,* for example by agreeing minimum standards of care and forming something akin to departmental quality circles to achieve them.

Conclusion

Cultures do not change overnight, particularly firmly entrenched ones. But the current radical reorganisation of the NHS affords a rare opportunity to try out new management styles. And there is good reason to try. Too often these days the name of Kafka is invoked to describe the atmosphere and the experience of working in the NHS.

In the rush to apply business principles to health care a major difference between hospitals and commercial companies must not be overlooked. Many people sacrifice money and status to work in the health service because they want to care for patients. That caring ethos is what sets the health service apart. Harnessing it for self-regulation through employee vigilance may well be the NHS's best hope for the future.

References

DoH (1993) *Guidance for Staff on Relations with the Public and the Media*. DoH, London.

HMSO (1992) *Report of the Committee of Inquiry into Complaints at Ashworth Special Hospital*. HMSO, London.

WINFIELD, M. (1990) *Minding Your Own Business: Self-Regulation and Whistleblowing in British Companies*. Social Audit, London.

8

Freedom of information

Diane Longley

> If information is the disinfectant of public life then freely available information is clearly an indispensable prerequisite of any democratic political system.
>
> (Birkinshaw *et al.*, 1990)

In 1974 Klein suggested that accountability within the health service should mean 'the acceptance of the responsibility to publicly explain and justify policies, to welcome rather than stifle discussion of priorities and objectives' as well as an 'awareness of and sensitivity to public needs and a willingness to remedy errors' (Klein, 1974, p. 365). He was advocating a far more open and user-responsive service. Such a service would require that decisions were not only justified and open to challenge *after* they have been taken but that the values reflected were those of the people most affected.

Inherently, accountability is evaluative. Its processes are the means by which the efficiency and effectiveness of an institution may be judged and ultimately the means by which legitimacy is lent to its conduct. But accountability is also a dynamic process, providing a vehicle for improvement. Without accountability, techniques for performance review and organisational assessment, the search for effective and good quality public services is likely to be impeded.

Accountability for the exercise of any public power has always been perplexing, often comprising a heterogeneous mix of fiscal, managerial, professional and public forms. Within the health service accountability is particularly tenuous. Essentially health care provision is rationed, requiring hard policy choices to be made about the selection of priorities, the allocation of resources and the availability of services. Inevitably trade-offs continually have to be made between costs, quality and access. Such policy decisions are often tacit rather than explicit, effected through extremely complex processes that involve a wide variety of participants and influences. At all levels within the health system decisions about the allocation of resources and the provision of services may be crucially affected by those who have access to the policy processes. Yet it is far from easy to map out the relative significant and shifting patterns of impact of the organisation's constituent groups; politicians, civil service, health authority managers and members, the medical professions and ancillaries and, of course, the consumer, not to mention any external pressures from the medical supply or pharmaceutical industries.

The central prerequisite for genuine accountability is openness, an accessibility to information that embraces all decision making from policy setting through implementation to monitoring. A commitment to openness is fundamental if any tendency to control or distort information is to be counteracted and issues are not to be prevented from being the subject of proper debate and so reducing the capacity for reasoned choices about priorities and resource distribution. Freedom of information is therefore essential.

But accountability and openness require more than a basic provision for access to information; they require the provision of mechanisms for the *actual generation* of information and its utilisation in the right form at the right time, so that the scope of options may be widened.

That same commitment also implies an obligation on the part of decision makers, whether managers or medical professionals, to give explanations and justifications for their activities. This not only assists the development of standards and principles but encourages more care and deliberation on the purposes of action, provides a basis for criticism and facilitates challenge to decisions that appear arbitrary. It is only through properly responsive processes of accountability that a clear picture of any service can emerge, defects be made apparent and any changing patterns of alliances highlighted. In this way opportunities can be provided for different interests and views to be brought to bear on practice and ultimately facilitate change.

Having set out the requirements for accountability generally in terms of information, the key question is whether these are currently being fulfilled within the NHS. Is there a high degree of accessibility to information? What kind of information is generated and to whom is it made available?

The patient

Let us begin from the perspective of the ultimate consumer of health care, the patient. The emphasis of the current NHS reorganisation is on individual choice and consumer sovereignty in the 'market'. By virtue of exercising greater choice in the provision of health services patients are meant to have a role in health care policy and quality assurance. However, the rhetoric is much stronger than the explanation of how this is actually exercised (Klein, 1989). It is now a well-rehearsed argument that there is little scope for the consumer to have any real choice at the point of entry into health care and the scarcity of information plays a part in this situation. Patients are to a great extent dependent on those who provide and purchase care on their behalf, so it is fundamental that this is regulated and patients are able to make their voice heard. The task of how best to get what is necessary to those who require it in an equitable as well as efficient manner incorporates the collective as well as individual perspective.

Some advances have been made. The Citizen's Charter states that the public is entitled to a greater degree of openness, with no secrecy about how public services are run, how much they cost and who carries responsibility. Full and accurate information should be given about the services provided and targets to be met, together with audited information about results achieved. This should be in a comparable form wherever possible. Those affected by services are to be consulted regularly and systematically to inform decisions about what should be provided and management will be expected to demonstrate that user views have been taken into account in setting standards.

The principles of the Citizen's and Patient's Charters are to be welcomed. The question is whether in practice they will deliver a better deal for the public and fulfil the opportunity to empower them as citizens or whether they will merely reinforce the public as consumer with only a limited capacity to influence policy decisions. Much depends on the quality of the mechanisms and procedures adopted to give substance to charter principles and the significance attached to them by those responsible for their implementation and monitoring.

Presently, throughout all levels of the NHS, the prevalent culture of closed decision making is proving difficult to dissipate. At central level, for example, objectives, strategy and finance are determined with the advice and support of the Policy Board which is chaired by the Secretary of State and whose members are drawn from government, the health service and industry. It is intended that the Board should be concerned with the overall pattern and balance of policy and assessment of its effectiveness, rather than any detailed formulation of specific plans. But the workings of the Policy Board and its relationship with the policy divisions of the Department of Health are something of a mystery. Although the membership of the Board is a mix of personnel and cultures which could produce some bargaining complexities, it is unlikely that their deliberations will ever reach public ears. Neither policy reports nor the responses of central management are made the subject of widespread scrutiny or comment. It is difficult, therefore, to estimate the extent to which the Board actually influences policy as opposed to legitimising what the Secretary of State for Health already has in mind. In order to be more effective and accountable for high level policy, the Board's debates need to be more transparent and procedures need to be put in place to facilitate input from a wider spectrum of interests.

In New Zealand, where reform of the health care system is also currently in progress, more consideration has been given to consultation and access to information at central management level, although some criticism can be made of consumer input into decision making locally under the new structure. A National Advisory Committee on Core Health and Disability Services was established by the New Zealand Minister of Health in March 1992 to receive independent advice on what health and disability support services should be purchased. It is under a duty to consult the public and make recommendations annually and periodically to the government. The Committee's first report was published in November 1992 and sets out current services, board priorities identified through consultation, letters and submissions, and guidelines for regional authorities to improve effectiveness, health outcomes and equity of access to some specific areas of service. New Zealand has had an Official Information Act since 1982, the provisions of which have been interpreted broadly and have lent support to the many substantial and innovative changes which are taking place throughout the management of public services.

Community health councils

One of the main avenues for dialogue about the provision of health services with the public at a more local level is, of course, the community health councils (CHC) (see Ch. 5). Although under the latest reorganisation the statutory duties of CHCs have remained unaltered, management executive guidance has introduced a number of key changes which affect CHC involvement in local health planning.

CHCs have a right to be consulted by the relevant district health authority (DHA) when a substantial development or a variation in services is contemplated. There are no provisions for CHCs to be consulted on health care issues on a wider regional or national basis, although some regional health authorities have on occasion involved CHCs in strategic planning. In addition, the Association of Community Health Councils in England and Wales (ACHCEW) regularly considers and submits responses to national policy documents to the Department of Health and the NHS Management Executive.

The provision for consultation suggests that there is an underlying intention that decisions should be taken in an open and reasoned manner, enabling differing interests to be taken into account before policy has become consolidated. Consultation procedures imply a commitment to openness and accountability. This view is reinforced in *Local Voices*, published by the Management Executive in 1992, which suggests ways in which to draw the views of the public into priority decisions. It emphasises the need for DHAs to develop *ongoing* involvement through dissemination of information and dialogue at all stages of the purchasing of health services. There are currently many innovative local initiatives building on these principles, but doubts must be expressed about their ability to influence policy in any other way but marginally. In practice consultation may result more in a process of exclusion than inclusion because of differential access to information and resources which enables privileged groups to set agendas and the terms of debate before dialogue actually begins (Harden and Lewis, 1986). Consequently the process of consultation, if not carefully structured and monitored, may simply perform a legitimising function rather than provide a channel for any real contribution in decision making. When responding to consultation a frequent complaint of CHCs and other interested parties is that they receive insufficient and such poor quality information about proposals that they are unable to make adequate comment, let alone suggest any viable alternatives.

Consultation procedures about applications for Trust status have been of equal concern. Such applications are subject to statutory public consultation which is undertaken by regional health authorities who then report the results to the Secretary of State. There is a duty to consult the CHC for the district in which the trust is to be located and other bodies whom the RHA considers to have an interest in the application or are directed to consult by the Health Minister. The government stated that it was important that trust applications are given wide publicity to ensure that all those who wish to make their views known have an opportunity to do so. However, meaningful consultation is reliant on the supply of sufficient information and mechanisms which are adequate to test relevant views. Similar criticisms to those made in regard to variations in services can be made of the trust application process. The period for consultation is only three months, a short time for a considered response to what are often only basic facts and from which financial details are omitted. Public meetings are left to the discretion of RHAs and trust applicants. It is significant that it is not until after the business plan has been developed and the application prepared that the statutory provision for consultation comes into play. Consultation is therefore conducted well after plans have crystallised and a great deal of time and energy have been expended. Amongst the key factors that trust applications are to focus on in order to obtain approval are the overall aims of the trust and the benefits to patients and the local community and the way in which services will be developed and quality assured. These are matters on which the public as consumers, either individually or collectively, might wish to comment and yet information is generally scant. It is also a matter of concern that trusts are under no duty to consult if they are considering the closure of a unit or a change in their activities.

As regards trust business generally, there is a perceived need for secrecy which runs contrary to the expectation of public accountability and openness. Although the government claims that trusts are opening themselves to unprecedented public scrutiny they are required to hold only one public meeting a year. Fewer than half of the trust boards have decided to meet in public more frequently. Although some arrange regular meetings with the CHC, only one in 15 allows a CHC representative into private board meetings. The majority have made other arrangements for communicating decisions to staff and the public. Selective provisions of information to the public does not make a trust accountable and concern about this has been expressed by the House of Commons Health Select Committee.

Current legislation is of little assistance to a greater degree of openness. In the UK the Public Bodies (Admission to Meetings) Act 1960 requires full regional and district health authority meetings to be open to the public. Notice of the time and place of meeting must be posted at the offices of the health authority at least three clear days before the meeting and the press must be supplied with a copy of the agenda and any further particulars necessary to indicate the nature of an item, on request. However, a health authority may exclude the public by resolution, whenever publicity would be prejudicial to the public interest by reason of the confidential nature of the business transacted or for special reasons. Legal requirements are thus limited and are rarely exceeded. In practice much health authority business is conducted without public scrutiny as exclusionary provisions are frequently interpreted broadly. The 1960 Act does not govern the conduct of business carried out in committees or subcommittees, which in many cases is extensive.

By contrast, in the USA not only does freedom of information legislation operate, but the 1977 Government in the Sunshine Act applies to all agencies of the executive branch of federal government and their subcommittees and advisory bodies. The Act provides that every part of every meeting shall be open to the public unless the subject matter is statutorily exempted. There are also requirements for records to be kept of closed meetings, procedures for public access to those records and rules for judicial review of any violation of the provisions of the Act.

District health authorities

Also of importance in the availability of information is the developing role of DHAs, that of 'champion of the people'. This has significant implications for public consultation about policy as DHAs are being encouraged to develop links with local resident and community groups. The current changes in both the structure and the function of DHAs could provide the opportunity to accommodate real consumer participation and the sharing of information rather than mere rhetorical acknowledgement and to redress the balance between management, medical professionals and the public. The consumer advocate function of DHAs is providing a challenge which entails changes to DHA philosophy and culture, which many health authorities are doing their best to meet. The means by which DHAs build up 'healthy alliances' are crucial to the establishment of public input into health care planning. The opportunity exists to develop effective representation and appraisal of all relevant interests and much depends on health authorities being prepared to be innovative about devising arrangements and open in their conduct.

In reality it is proving extremely difficult for health authorities to adopt a role of reconciling the potentially varying views about what is needed in the locality. There is an indication that purchaser buying patterns do not reflect listings of priorities and objectives which result from consultation exercises. For example, mental health, care of the elderly and coronary care frequently feature as areas for funding and development, but come very low in actual spending in signed contracts. It seems that there is some reluctance on the part of district health authorities to make hard choices and there remains a tendency to satisfy as many interests as possible. Responsiveness to public needs does not yet appear to be uppermost as purchasers face competing demands from the centre, region, providers and the community. The point is that the influences underlying those compromises are still not explicit and there is a lack of information about the growth of any informal, and therefore unaccountable, alliances which might develop to protect mutual interests between purchasers and providers.

Avoidance of the latter requires a strong commitment to open decision making and broadened access to data. One of the key factors is to ensure that information is available at a time and in a form that optimises its usefulness but this is currently constrained by both managerial and operational policy. The latest reforms have largely failed to grasp the opportunity to enhance participation in health policy by the public and their representatives and statutory consultation procedures remain minimal and for the most part marginally effective. The classic case of too little, too late.

Public effectiveness in countering manager or provider perspectives is likely to continue towards tokenism unless supported by an institutional framework that is procedurally structured to ensure that all interests are properly taken into account and issues are not kept from open discussion. Health care is without doubt a political issue in its true sense and any legitimate analysis of its provision necessitates informed debate on all perspectives. The networks being developed by DHAs currently rely more on goodwill than any clear structural guidance. Changes need to be made as regards the powers, organisation and available resources for consumer input. As ACHCEW have pointed out, for the public to be empowered and participate fully in health care decisions it is essential that there is consistent access to information about the quality of local services and available options.

Monitoring quality

In recent years there has been a steadily increasing awareness of the need to monitor and appraise the quality of all public services. Although fuelled largely by the desire to contain costs and attain value for money, many major initiatives have produced some indepth debates about indicators for assessing quality of service and consumer need (Pollitt, 1986). Within the health care field the difficulties of providing quality services are a major issue. The inevitable tension which exists between the attainment or maintenance of quality and fiscal issues gives rise to legitimate and pressing matters which involve both financing and accountability processes.

Monitoring quality is a problematic process which needs to be carefully planned and executed. A whole spectrum of quality issues exist which involve individual and collective matters and which range from technical matters through the activities of the medical profession and management, where responsibilities overlap, to the quality of outcomes. Needless to say, this requires a substantial investment in resources and information gathering and may create difficulties with 'ownership' of that information.

Resource management

A prime example is the Resource Management Initiative (RMI) which was first introduced on an experimental basis in 1986. When first established the programme was intended principally to be about altering the attitude of clinicians towards taking account of resource utilisation and encouraging closer teamwork amongst medical professionals and other managers in resource management. Before any decisions were to be taken about implementation in the rest of the health service a progress review of the first six sites was to have been published. However, events of the latest health service reform overtook a full analysis of the initiative. In order for contracting to work effectively as the vehicle which now underpins the provision of health services, a comprehensive means of accounting for the utilisation and costs of resources had to be established. Consequently investment in resource management systems is now a national initiative despite doubts raised about its effect on clinical practice and growing awareness of the financial consequences of its implementation. But considerable investment in the development of financial and resource information systems can only be justified if it can be demonstrated that an increase in benefits flows from their imposition. The cost of acquisition of information has to be balanced against improvements in quality and efficiency in the provision of services. There are presently serious difficulties with the implementation of resource management in terms of technical accounting, the availability of the necessary information technology and confusion about control and possession of the system. It has been pointed out that information systems take on different forms according to the balance of concerns represented during the process of development and two extreme perspectives of resource management can be identified; one is clinically led, the other is financial management oriented (Coombs and Cooper, 1990; Packwood *et al.*, 1991). Emphasis on the latter can result in insufficient consideration being given to medical evaluation of respective treatments. Furthermore, it could result in a lack of attention being given to cost dumping, where savings in one area of health care are more than offset by additional costs in others. The main concern is that shifts in practice can be attempted through the development of information systems which fail to articulate the fact that particular sorts of information are privileged and serve to reinforce specific and often potent perspectives about what the aims of health care are or should be (Coombs and Cooper, 1990, p. 9).

However, the gains for the health services arising from the implementation and processes of resource management could be immense in relation to financial, professional and public accountability. Neither should its potential benefit for health service and organisational quality be underestimated. Much has been learned already. Resource management can enable services to be genuinely managed, promote collaboration and combine accountability for decisions about the allocation of resources, their management and planning and review of services into 'a coherent whole' (Packwood *et al.*, 1991, p. 75).

Properly considered and *openly* operated resource management can offer a chance for management, medical professionals and consumers to plan health services on a more rational basis by supplying evidence of use and needs and highlighting requirements for change in the deployment of resources. It can therefore provide an opportunity for genuine local decision making. Much depends on the theme of this chapter; the gathering of necessary information, its interpretation and the use to which it is put. This does not automatically mean an investment in the development of high technology data collection. Many examples of the successes of resource management have arisen not from the provision of sophisticated data, but from the improved capacity and means to agree a strategy (Packwood *et al.*, 1991, p. 158).

Resource management could fail to reach its full potential if information gathering is restricted to cost effectiveness and excludes other important elements. It has not yet had the impact on the relationship between providers and the consumer that it could have, although it has resulted in some internal adjustments between different interest groups within the NHS. Attitudes need to be changed, trust built and an integrated system developed in which information is shared. Without freedom of information opportunities for accountability are lost. Only if all those concerned with its exercise can see clearly and openly the benefits of resource management, by rendering visible what are now often tacit features of health care provision, will it be able to develop into a successful social resource for improving and assuring the quality of health services and the efficiency of its provision.

Medical audit

Similar concerns about the accessibility of information and the use to which it is put exist in relation to medical audit. Medical audit is part of the overall package of resource control and is central to the programme to enhance overall quality of care. It is described as a systematic and critical analysis of the quality of medical care, including the procedures used for diagnosis and treatment, the use of resources and the resulting outcome and quality of life for the patient. A requirement to participate in audit is included in consultants' contracts and general practitioner terms of service and it is intended that every doctor and medical team should take part in regular systematic audit.

Because medical audit is regarded as requiring specialised knowledge of current medical practice and access to medical records the approach that has been taken is firmly based on the principle of peer review. But as management have the task of monitoring the use of resources they have been given the responsibility of ensuring that an effective system of audit is developed. The form of audit and the frequency of review have generally been a matter of negotiation between management and medical professionals locally and may give rise to some tension as to which group is to lead the scheme.

The results of audit in respect of individual patients and doctors remain confidential at all times, but general results are made available to local management in order to satisfy them that the appropriate remedial action is taken where problems have been experienced. If management are not satisfied that resources are being used to the best effect they can request the district audit advisory committee (DAAC) to initiate an independent audit which may take the form of a peer review carried out by clinicians from outside the district or a joint management and professional appraisal of a particular service.

A central function of the DAAC is to plan and monitor a comprehensive programme for audit which is expected to incorporate the views of patients. Each committee will produce an annual forward plan which will specify the methods to be used and the frequency of audit for each clinical team. It will also specify a rolling programme under which the treatment of particular conditions is to be reviewed collectively by relevant clinicians. This is also expected to include longer term results involving collaboration with primary care. The committee is expected to produce an annual report on the previous year's activity which details procedures used and services covered together with actual or recommended follow-up action where the means of improving quality or efficiency of care have been identified. It has been suggested that relevant parts of both the forward plan and the annual report could be made available to other health authorities who are considering placing contracts within the district, but there is *no* mention of any further dissemination of audit information.

The provisions for medical audit have been widely welcomed by professionals and consumer organisations, although there is some criticism. Taken at face value the purpose of medical audit is to evaluate the quality of care, but a closer look appears to suggest a lack of commitment on the part of government to develop adequate measures for actual monitoring and improvement of quality. This arises from a lack of clarity about the conception of audit with which NHS management is intended to operate. It has been pointed out that audits are not just descriptions, as the values underlying them not only influence responses to evaluation criteria but also influence awareness of both alternatives and priorities. As with resource management there is a feeling that the primary concern is cost effectiveness, which is evidenced by a confusion between medical audit and monitoring for value for money in NHS literature. Both are necessary and legitimate processes, but they are different in nature. In negotiating and regulating contracts for care, health authorities need to take account of medical audit and arrangements alongside those of other types of overall quality and costs.

Like resource management medical audit requires a significant investment not only financially but in terms of clinicians' time and energies, as well as that of support staff, to ensure the necessary information is available. At present information systems are often no more than rudimentary; it takes long consideration and time to develop and refine measures into useful medical and management tools. It is important that the systems that develop do not do so independently of one another and are able to link information so that more complete evidence on quality of the continuation of care between primary, secondary and related services can be provided. Good examples of audit need to be documented, evaluated and then disseminated so that others can learn and build on proven methods and utilise findings.

The various means of quality assurance undoubtedly supplement and complement one another. But for several reasons doubts persist that the schemes which are being promoted are adequate to provide true review and monitoring of quality. In the first instance there is an overall preoccupation with the quantification of results. Information on outcomes needs to be considered alongside data on activity levels, cost and length of stay to demonstrate that improvements are real and that increases in activity or quantity are not at the expense of quality. Otherwise an increase in readmission and complication rates might result. But there is as yet an inability to generate information on outcomes. Much of what is available is still of questionable accuracy and hence of marginal use. Doubts must therefore be expressed about the utility of information to be published in health authority league tables. These seem likely to indicate comparison of supply costs or waiting times of which limited use can be made by the public where their capacity for choice is inherently restricted.

In the USA there is a much deeper commitment to reducing the above deficiencies. The federal government funds research to generate information on the definition of quality and examine quality evaluation tools. Recently support has been provided for an examination of the relationship between variations in practice and quality and between quality of care and health outcomes in several areas of clinical activity. In addition, peer review organisations (PRO) provide a primary means of obtaining evaluative information on health care quality as they receive and generate a vast quantity of data. Although PRO regulations limit public release of information they do permit disclosure of quality data regarding health care institutions. Furthermore, a majority of states have now passed legislation to compel release of information collected by providers (Jost, 1988).

In summary, access to information is necessary for our knowing where our health service has come from, why it is the way it is, where it is going, what its aspirations are and what forces are influencing and shaping fundamental choices. We need first to understand our expectations for our health systems in order to work towards a realisation or adjustment of those expectations by setting realistic standards for improvement. The very nature of accountability dictates that the initiative must be taken by those who question the decisions being taken. Currently, that initiative is not held by the public. Health authorities decide what information will be made available, in what form and also decide on the form any consultation should take. In the absence of freedom of information there is no way of verifying what we are being told. Whilst health authorities are bodies with a potential for generating debate and testing critical assumptions as well as providing opportunities to make creative use of planning evaluation, because of their many competing interests and allegiances they cannot be relied upon to respond effectively to public concerns.

Ultimately there is a need for an *independent* generation of information. Currently there is too extensive a focus on single events and single settings rather than episodes or continuity of care. The result is that decisions are often taken in isolation or ignorance of other factors and policy at all levels is ill-founded. There is no oversight group with the breadth of vision or independence to analyse data from every possible source, identify barriers to improvement of services and make recommendations which can be fed into policy processes. Without such information becoming available and being shared, overall health gains are unlikely.

The salient lesson is that information, the way it is collected, for what purpose, the scope of its dissemination and its incorporation into policy all need to be seriously and carefully considered before any further investment in time and resources is made. As the quality of information ultimately affects the quality of service there is an urgent need for the development of an information strategy backed by freedom of information legislation.

Access to personal information

The discussion so far in this chapter has focused on the wider availability of information for policy decisions. This section briefly looks at access to information of a more personal nature, that held on medical records.

Access to information held in health records has had a contentious history not least because any wide access to information could lead to serious infringements of privacy and breaches of confidentiality if not carefully regulated. That aside, patient representative groups and the Campaign for Freedom of Information have fought long and hard for patients to have a right of access to their own medical records. But a number of attempts to move in this direction have been strongly resisted by much of the medical profession who have tended to take a rather paternalistic and narrow view of the amount and kind of medical information patients should receive. In addition little support has been lent to requests for access by the courts who have frequently taken a deferential stand to the arguments put forward by doctors and their representative bodies. But there are a number of circumstances in which a patient may seek information about their health held on medical records, such as in preparation or in the course of litigation or complaint or when seeking a second opinion and deciding on a course of action.

In the UK the response to calls for access to personal information has been piecemeal. In some respects legislation has not gone as far as some jurisdictions, in others it has gone further. The principal statutes relating to health are the Data Protection Act 1984, the Access to Medical Reports Act 1988 and the Access to Health Records Act 1991.

Since 1987 patients have been able to request a copy of any information held about them on computer under the Data Protection Act 1984. However, the Data Protection (Subject Access Modification) (Health) Order regulations modified the basic provisions of the Act to provide that access can be refused to patients where it would be likely to cause serious harm to the physical or mental health of the patient or lead to identification of another person to whom the information might relate. The Act requires that a request for access must be made in writing and accompanied by the appropriate fee.

Although this was a significant improvement the requirement for a fee in some cases has proved something of a deterrent. Additionally many health records remain uncomputerised and the Act does not therefore apply in those circumstances. In fact, it has been argued that the reluctance of the medical profession to approve access to medical files has acted as a positive disincentive to computerise records (Brazier, 1992). Difficulties can also exist for the patient who seeks to challenge the withholding of information under the Act, as the common law has generally given little support to patients in such instances.

Until recently the only access patients had to records held manually was provided by the Access to Medical Files Act 1988 which allows access in certain circumstances to any medical report which has been supplied for the purpose of employment or insurance. It gives no right of access to medical files generally. The regulations and access provisions of this Act are to some extent more restrictive than their counterparts in other common law jurisdictions (Birkinshaw *et al.*, 1990). The patient's consent to a medical report being sought must be obtained by any employer or insurance company. If the doctor giving the medical report is not the patient's general practitioner the Act does not apply. Similar exemptions to those of the Data Protection Act apply and there is provision for an application to be made to the court if access is wrongly refused. A reasonable fee may be charged for a copy of the medical report.

Despite government support for a patient's right of access to manually held medical files, it was not until 1990 that the Access to Health Records Act was introduced into Parliament. The Act, which covers both public and private sector, applies to manual health records held by or on behalf of a health professional and allows for inspection and copying by the applicant. It also requires an explanation to be given for any information that is unintelligible. However, the provisions apply only to records compiled since November 1991 when the Act came into force. There are, of course, exclusions which follow the general pattern already described. Although initially exclusionary principles may appear reasonable, they can be used by health authorities and doctors to deny access unnecessarily. The patient may have considerable difficulty in applying under the Act to the court for disclosure of information because the common law confers no right of access and tends to give undue weight to the judgements of the medical profession.

Applications for access outside the three principal acts mentioned may be considered by the courts in limited circumstances. For example, the Supreme Court Act 1981 (ss. 33, 34) makes provision for access to medical files where litigation has been commenced or is being seriously contemplated. But even this Act may restrict disclosure as complex questions of ownership of information and even questions of who owned the paper on which records are written have at times thwarted applicants (Brazier, 1992, p. 63).

What is really needed is a change of attitude to patient access of information and reduction of paternalism in the medical profession. This can come only from well-considered support of legislative provisions by the courts. Doctors have on the whole not welcomed patient access to their medical records because they feel that it inhibits their capacity to be frank. But this can in turn lead to irregular and inadequate records being kept. One of the most repeated criticisms by the Health Service Commissioner in annual reports is the poor quality of medical records. Ultimately this affects the quality of overall care.

In New Zealand hospitals and health boards were brought under the 1982 Official Information Act a number of years ago. Most importantly the Act relates to *information*, not just documents, and includes what is in a doctor's mind as much as what is committed to the patient's *written* record. This has meant that recollections have had to be put into writing at the insistence of the Chief Ombudsman. Exemptions to access are similar to those in the UK where disclosure might prejudice a person's physical or mental well-being or identify a third party. Although the Act does not apply to private hospitals or practitioners, a fact which has been the source of some confusion, it has resulted in changes to professional attitudes.

Conclusion

Health is at the centre of any sustainable social and economic activity. The pursuit of health, whether on an individual or collective basis, is about communication and cooperation. That pursuit requires the availability of information. As the focus of health moves away from collective community health approaches towards medical procedures and individual patient care, ways need to be found to recreate an environment which supports community involvement and action in health care decisions. We need to consider how this could affect information, the control of which can give inequitable advantages. The sharing of information between public agencies and between those agencies and the public is already limited. For the new pro-market perspectives to function effectively the consumer must have knowledge of health status and the competence of providers as well as relevant treatment and available options. Lack of knowledge is currently a persistent problem. Commercial sensitivity and professional attitudes can prevent the sharing and dissemination of critical information. Changes in the availability of information cannot be left to good will and freedom of information needs to become part of the life-sustaining circulatory system of our health services.

References

BIRKINSHAW, P., HARDEN, I. AND LEWIS, N. (1990) *Government by Moonlight: The Hybrid Parts of the State.* Unwin Hyman, London.

BRAZIER, M. (1992) *Medicine, Patients and the Law,* 2nd ed., Penguin Books, Harmondsworth.

COOMBS, R. AND COOPER, R. (1990) *Accounting for Patients? Information Technology and the NHS White Paper.* Paper 10. Manchester Centre for Research on Organisations, Management and Technical Change, UMIST, Manchester.

HARDEN, I. AND LEWIS, N. (1986) *The Noble Lie: The British Constitution and the Rule of Law.* Hutchinson, London.

JOST, T. (1988) The necessary and proper role of regulation to assure the quality of care. *Houston Law Review* **25**, 525.

KLEIN, R. (1974) Accountability in the health service. *Political Quarterly* **42**, 364.

KLEIN, R. (1989) *The Politics of the NHS,* 2nd ed. Longman, Harlow.

PACKWOOD, T., KEEN J. and BUXTON, M. (1991) *Hospitals in Transition: The Resource Management Experiment.* Open University Press, Milton Keynes.

POLLITT, C. (1986) Beyond the managerial model: the case for broadening performance assessment in government and public services. *Financial Accountability and Management* **2(3)**, 155.

9

Whistleblowing in American health care

Jean McHale

At a time when health care issues are increasingly debated at an international level some comparison of approaches to whistleblowing in other jurisdictions might be pertinent. This chapter seeks to examine how far health care professionals who believe it is their duty to blow the whistle on poor care standards are protected in the United States compared with their British counterparts. The comparison with the United States is particularly instructive for several reasons. In the United States there has always been considerable emphasis on protecting free speech – a right recognised in the Constitution. There is an on-going debate on issues of ethics, informed consent and patient rights in the United States. Medical decision-making has come under greater public scrutiny in both courtroom and committee, and fundamental questions of ethical importance, such as informed consent and decisions about forgoing life-saving treatment have been investigated at the highest level by bodies such as the President's Commission on Bioethics (Capron, 1988). In some situations the health care professional may decide to blow the whistle as advocate – safeguarding the rights of the patient. In the United Kingdom much of the controversy about whistleblowing concerns nursing practice. It must not be forgotten that much of the dialogue surrounding the nurse as patient advocate originated in the United States. The nurse as patient advocate may believe that it is part of her duty to speak out when patient care is at risk. Finally, the emphasis on private health care in the States has meant that patients dissatisfied with the care given to them have, in effect, voted with their feet.

A brief overview of the US health care system reveals many ways in which concerns over poor care standards might be raised and legal mechanisms which safeguard the whistleblower. But closer scrutiny reveals the position to be far less satisfactory. Much of the debate regarding patient rights is at the level of high policy as opposed to the practical questions of ensuring that these rights are respected on the ground. While the role of nurse as patient advocate has been recognised that does not mean that it has received anything approaching total acceptance. If the nurse does decide to act as an advocate she may find herself in a difficult position. In a case reported by Winslow (1984) a nurse was present when a surgical resident in a hospital made a mistake during a tracheotomy operation and as a result severed the patient's carotid artery. The patient bled to death. Despite this the nurse was cautioned that before she reported this case she should get herself a lawyer! The freedom to vote with your feet by going to another health care practitioner has been limited by the development of care contracts (Friedson, 1987; Raffel, 1989). Increasingly, insured patients are required to take their care from organisations such as Health Maintenance Organisations – groups of practitioners with whom their insurers have an agreement.

With less flexibility for patients it is of increasing importance to ensure that the standard of care given by health care providers is adequately monitored and that abuses do not occur. The health care professional is in many ways best placed to observe any drop in standards. But if standards do slide what can she do? In the first part of the chapter I discuss some of the various ways in which poor care standards can be identified and concerns addressed within the health care system. The second part examines some of the mechanisms of redress provided in law where whistleblowing does occur. This chapter is not a totally comprehensive coverage of all whistleblowing issues raised in the United States.

Regulating health care

In the United States the provision of health care is monitored through a number of mechanisms. Legislation requires that hospitals be licensed. The scope of these licensing laws extends from hospital safety to patient care. Where patients are cared for in nursing homes their care may be regulated by statute. Nursing homes have to be licensed and abuses should be reported to licensing authorities (Raffel, 1989).

Joint commission

A major force in monitoring standards of care is the Joint Commission on Accreditation of Hospitals. This organisation was established by the American College of Physicians, American Hospital Association and American Medical Association in 1952. The committee investigates hospitals, accrediting those which provide quality care. They also accredit numerous other health care organisations. Accreditation is in practice crucial since hospitals need to show that they are accredited in order to reimburse claims for treatment given to patients made under the public insurance schemes, Medicare and Medicaid. In addition the very fact of accreditation may be sufficient for a hospital to comply with a state's licensing requirements. As part of their accrediting role Joint Commission Committees undertake visits to hospitals during which meetings are held with staff giving an opportunity for complaints to be made (Friedson, 1987).

Accredited hospitals must establish committees to review care. The Committees are usually composed of hospital staff members including a doctor, a nurse, an administrator, and a medical technologist. They are responsible for reviewing and evaluating the professional qualifications and professional practices of other staff members.

Patients treated in accredited hospitals have the right to make complaints to the institution and or someone may complain on the patient's behalf (42 US Code S 13.20 c(3)(a)). The first port of call for such complaints is likely to be the state health department and then if a grievance remains matters may be taken to the Joint Commission. It is possible that a health care professional may bring complaints on the patient's behalf – though in practice this is unlikely. There appears to be a divergence of opinion over the effectiveness of Joint Commission reviews. It has been argued that:

> neither the way committee reviews were conducted nor their findings were subjected to very close or critical scrutiny and accreditation requirements left great leeway in their mode of operation.
>
> (Friedson, 1987)

But other commentators, such as Raffel (1989), identify areas in which the Joint Commission has instituted improvements in care. Their influence can be seen in the pressure placed upon hospital doctors to keep patient records up to date and ensure that regular reviews are undertaken during pathology reports on all tissues removed in surgery to check that unnecessary surgery is not being undertaken. An independent body of the nature of the Joint Commission reviewing all types of hospital care both state and private might provide a useful mechanism for scrutiny in the UK but it would need to be accompanied by a wide-ranging review of hospital complaints and would also require acceptance by both public and private sector health care.

Patient representatives

There has been a major debate on patient rights in the USA and the impact of this debate can be seen in individual hospitals. States have enacted declarations of patient rights and legislation stipulates that these be brought to the attention of patients. For example, in New Jersey not only does legislation provide that patients are entitled to be given a summary of their rights but hospitals are also required to provide a designated staff member to deal with grievances and give the number of government agencies to whom complaint can be made. Certain US hospitals have appointed a complaints officer (a patient representative or patient ombudsman) to work within the hospital. Though employed by the hospital this officer acts independently of the hospital. Patients and staff can bring their concerns and the officer will investigate the grievance and, where this is substantiated, raise the matter with the hospital management. The types of issues scrutinised include medical service, quality of care, risk management, inter-personal skills, communication, and access issues. Good relations between the patient representative and the hospital management promote the redress of grievances. But in an extreme case if a grievance has not been met then a patient representative may feel that it is his or her duty to go outside the institution and complain in public. This may provide an effective means for addressing those concerns which may otherwise lead clinical staff members to blow the whistle.

There is also a danger in expecting too much from the patient representative. The patient representative's role is limited to considering grievances which arise in the individual institution. The fact that the patient representative is an employee of the hospital might inhibit persons from coming forward because he or she may be perceived as lacking the necessary degree of independence. However her role may be strengthened if she is a member of the national association of patient representatives and/or one of the state societies of patient representatives.

At present in the UK there is a movement towards establishing patient representatives within hospitals. Development of this role may encourage increasing openness in medical practice. However too much cannot be expected instantly of such a person. The role requires acceptance by professionals, by patients and hospital authorities and the person would have to tread a careful line to ensure that independence is maintained. Consultation between representatives from different hospitals would be crucial. This role could perhaps link in with that of a general body with the task of monitoring health care standards such as the Joint Commission.

Insurance agencies

While there has been an increasing movement in the UK towards the provision of private medical care funded by insurance the situation is still considerably different from that in the United States. US health care is funded through health insurance with physicians' fees being reimbursed by insurers. Patients are insured through their employment. Those who are unwaged may be covered by the public insurance schemes, Medicare and Medicaid. Care standards are to a certain extent monitored by insurers. When insurers examine claims for reimbursement they consider matters such as the appropriateness of treatment plans. But while they may review standards of care it is important to remember that these organisations are not solely influenced by considerations of quality. For example, in the private sector Private Utilisation Review Corporations consider claims for reimbursement, but their effectiveness may be somewhat diluted by the fact that their primary aim is the reduction of costs (Moran and Wood, 1993). They have succeeded in this; estimates have been given that they have cut hospital expenditure by 11.9% and medical expenditure by 8.3%.

Claims for reimbursement under the public sector insurers Medicare and Medicaid are handled by Peer Review Organizations (PRO). These have the task of examining treatment given in ambulatory care and in hospitals, questioning whether the treatment given was appropriate in the circumstances. Contracts are awarded to teams to undertake this work with preference given to physician-dominated teams. If malpractice or poor standards of care come to the attention of PRO they may raise their concerns at state level and ultimately may make recommendations to the Department of Health and Human Services which has the power to ban doctors from treating Medicare patients (Rosenthall, 1988). Evidence suggests that the PRO have been effective in at least some areas of health care with, for example a drop in unnecessary surgery due to sloppy diagnosis (Raffel, 1989).

Ethics committees

Bad or unethical practice may be uncovered when cases are considered by an institutional ethics committee (what would in the UK be called a hospital ethics committee) (McCall Smith, 1990). This is a multi-disciplinary committee established within a hospital. The committee considers both issues regarding the treatment of individual patients such as whether a life support system should be removed and questions such as the policy on the use of 'do not resuscitate' orders (Gibson and Kushner, 1986). The committees have been given a high profile and their decisions have been reviewed and approved by the courts (*Re Quinlan* 355 A.2d 647 (NJ 1976)), and professional organisations such as the American Nursing Association have actively encouraged involvement in such committees. In the UK there are no such committees, though writers such as McCall Smith have argued strongly in favour of them. Such committees may have their merits but as an antidote to poor care standards it is unlikely that they would play an extensive role. While institutional ethics committees play a valuable role in subjecting health care decisions to public scrutiny they are not a complaints monitoring body, unlike the Joint Commission. Only a handful of treatment decisions come to their attention. Institutional ethics committees are really forums for debating many of the controversial ethical questions relating to treatment.

Professional bodies

One method of dealing with abuses in standards of care rather than going fully public is for the matter to be referred to one of the professional regulatory agencies. As in the UK health care professionals are regulated by professional bodies. In the United States each state has a medical licensure board and one of their tasks is to discipline those physicians found to be incompetent or who have taken part in 'unprofessional conduct'. Health care professionals may make complaints about fellow professionals to these boards (Jost et al, 1993).

But, while research on complaints made to disciplinary bodies is still in its infancy, it appears that disciplinary action is rarely taken in response to complaints. One reason behind this appears to be because the statutes establishing offences either fail to define disciplinary offences or where they do the definition given is unsatisfactory. For example, the California Board of Medical Quality Assurance can only review specific complaints against a doctor. But before a doctor's licence can be revoked statute requires that a pattern of gross negligence by the doctor is shown. As Moran and Wood (1993) comment, it would be difficult to establish a case unless a large number of specific complaints are lodged against the doctor. Bringing disciplinary action may also take a long time. In Michigan cases may take up to two and a half years (Moran and Wood, 1993). In addition physicians who are licensed to practise in more than one state may simply move from one state to another (Rosenthall, 1992).

Procedures are now being tightened and more rigorous reporting of malpractice has become mandatory. A national practitioner data bank was set up in April 1990 providing a central computer register of information concerning disciplinary actions. However, much is still to be done. As Rosenthall (1992) has commented: 'The chronic problems of lack of resources, limitations on excessive authority, poor information sharing, lack of standards . . . still seriously hamper their activities'.

Reliance on professional bodies as a means of tackling the problems which cause whistleblowing is also unlikely to be a successful strategy in the UK. Leaving aside considerations of the practical problems of establishing complaints, professional bodies can only address a limited number of issues which come before them. They do not provide a proper forum for identifying and monitoring standards of care on a more general basis.

While mechanisms for scrutiny do exist in the United States they are disparate and criticism has been made of their operation. If health care professionals believe that immediate action is required and that existing channels for complaint are inadequate they may feel that the only way is to make known their concerns outside the institution to the media or another body. But they face the danger that disclosure may lead to dismissal.

Legal protection for whistleblowers

Common law – the public interest exception

Protection has been given to whistleblowers both in the common law courts and through the enactment of statutes at state and federal level. However, while a cursory glance reveals a large number of statutes and cases in which whistleblowers have been protected, closer examination reveals that the actual protection given is very incomplete and whistleblowers may face difficulties in bringing a claim.

United States employment law is based upon a 'hire and fire' system in which an employer is able to dismiss his employee without having to give a good reason. In recent years the draconian nature of this rule has been curtailed. The courts have been prepared to assume a covenant of good faith and fair dealing within the contract of employment. In some cases employees have succeeded in showing that the action for which they were dismissed was in the public interest and the employer has been held liable in the tort of abusive discharge (Howard, 1988).

Courts in over half of all US states now recognize a public policy exception to the termination-at-will rule. The exception has been used to protect health care workers who have complained about deficiencies in care (Haynes, 1988). Take, for example, the case of Sandra Bardenilla. Bardenilla resigned as nursing supervisor of a hospital ICU unit after the hospital failed to follow up on her attempts to formulate policies for removal of respiratory and nutritional support in her unit (Fry, 1989; Steinbock, 1983). A doctor gave instructions that a patient should be given care which she regarded as being both unethical and potentially illegal. The patient later died. Ms Bardenilla discussed her concern with the nursing director of the hospital but was told to be quiet and to apologise to the doctor. She resigned, brought a suit for wrongful termination of employment and was awarded $114 000 damages.

But while a public interest defence has been recognised an employee may find it difficult to establish that his own action is in the public interest. In *Pierce v. Ortho Pharmaceuticals* (84 NJ 1980) Dr Pierce joined Ortho Pharmaceuticals as associate director of medical research. She refused to proceed with tests on humans of a new drug, Loperamide. The drug was for the relief of acute and chronic diarrhoea and it had a high saccharine content to conceal its very bitter taste. A body of scientific opinion believed that saccharine caused cancer. The research team said that the drug should be reformulated and the saccharine level reduced. However, after the management applied pressure a number of the researchers in the team decided to go ahead with the trial. Dr Pierce refused and was accused by her employers of irresponsibility and lack of judgement. She was first taken off all therapeutic drug projects and then was later told that she was to be demoted with restrictions placed on the research associates she could work with. Dr Pierce resigned claiming that she had suffered damage to her professional reputation and disruption of her career. At first instance, the New Jersey Superior Court judge ruled in favour of Ortho upholding the principle that an employee can be fired at will. Dr Pierce appealed. The appellate division of the New Jersey Superior court reversed the decision and sent the case back for trial 'on all of the issues raised by the pleadings'. However, the court took a restrictive approach to public policy. It said that exceptions to the employment-at-will doctrine must be restricted to cases which involved truly significant matters of clear and well-defined public policy. The New Jersey Superior Court ruled that Dr Pierce's judgement and that of the company were simply at variance and that professional ethics was not an issue. They therefore upheld Ortho's claim.

Dr Pierce experienced difficulty in obtaining alternative employment, a common problem faced by whistleblowers. However, the disclosure did have implications for the drug trial. The company did not proceed to test the drug stating that the formula was 'inconvenient for patients'.

An employee will not necessarily be held to have acted in the public interest even if the conduct which formed the basis of allegations was outlawed by statute. In *Maus v. National Living Centers* (633 SW 2d 674 (Texa Civ App 1982)) the plaintiff, a nurse aid, was employed at the defendant's nursing home. He was sacked because he frequently complained to his superiors that patients were being neglected. One complaint concerned the refusal of the director of nursing at the home to call a doctor for a patient who had suffered a stroke. The plaintiff had administered CPR and kept the patient alive for several days before the patient's death. The law in the state of Texas provided that it was an offence to fail to report abuse or neglect of nursing home patients. While recognising that other jurisdictions had limited the right of an employer to terminate-at-will, the court nevertheless rejected the plaintiff's claim and regarded itself bound by the 'terminable-at-will' doctrine.

A narrow approach was also taken in *Lampe v. Presbyterian Medical Centre* (41 Colo App 465, 590 P 2d 513 (1978)). The contract of a nurse was terminated after she complained that changes in hospital staffing patterns put patient care at risk. The court held that no specific statute protected her from being fired. They rejected the argument that because her actions were in furtherance with the state Nurse Practice Acts, she should be protected.

Health care professionals may claim that their ethical code required them to speak out in the interests of patients. But that does not guarantee that a court will find that they acted in the public interest. In *Wartho v. Toms River Community Memorial Hospital* (199 NJ Super 8 App Div (1985)) the court held that despite the fact that a nurse's ethical code allowed the plaintiff to refuse to administer treatment believed to be incompatible with human dignity, she could not rely upon the code as the basis of her claim that the dismissal was unlawful. The code benefited only individuals and was not actionable (but compare the earlier case of *Kalman v. Grand Union Co* (183 NJ Super App Div (1982)). The courts have not been willing to support claims of persons who have been dismissed after they have complained internally within an organisation. (*Geary v. US Steel Corporation* 456 Pa 171 319 p 2ND (1974)); *Mud v. Hoffman Homes for Youth* (374 Pa Super 522, 543, A.2ND (1988)); *Zaniecki v. P. A. Bergner and Co.* (143 11 App 3d 668, 493, N.E.2d 419 (1986)).

Rongine (1985) has suggested that the situation could be improved by the introduction of legislation defining what amounts to the public interest. But obtaining agreement as to what amounts to the public interest may be difficult. The scope of protection given at present in US law illustrates how the problem can vary quite dramatically. Some statutes only protect disclosures where a violation of law has taken place while others protect disclosures made in situations in which it is reasonably believed that a violation had taken place. Frequently statutes provide that protection will only be given if the disclosure is to a defined person or official.

The whistleblowing employee may be in a stronger position if the employment relationship is governed by a collective bargaining agreement and he has resort to arbitrators appointed under such an agreement (Malin, 1983). These agreements frequently require an employer to have 'just cause' to discharge employees. One advantage in having your case heard by an arbitrator is that arbitrators are far more likely to order reinstatement (Furrow *et al.*, 1981). An illustration is provided by the case of *Olympia Memorial Hospital* (1981-Lab Arb (C.C.H.) s 8059 (1980)). Three nurses expressed their concerns to their superior regarding the competence of the director of nursing. The employer said that these charges were false and that the complainants had disrupted morale and interfered with the ordinary operation of the hospital. Arbitrators, however, awarded reinstatement stressing that the complaints had been made in good faith and suggested that had the nurses stayed silent this would have compromised their responsibility to their patients.

Constitutional protection

The United States Constitution has been used to protect those employees who have spoken publicly about inadequate standards. Whistleblowers have claimed that retaliatory action taken against them is unlawful because it contravenes the free speech right. The First Amendment of the United States constitution provides that:

> Congress shall make no law respecting an establishment of religion or prohibiting the free exercise thereof; or abridging the freedom of speech or of the press; or the right of the people peaceably to assemble and to petition the Government for a redress of grievances.

In *Rafferty v. Philadelphia Psychiatric Centre* the federal court reinstated a nurse discharged because of criticism of patient care which appeared in public news articles. The First Amendment has also been applied by federal appellate courts to private employers (*Nousel v. Nationwide Insurance Company*, 721 F.2d 894 (CA 3193)). However, there are difficulties in reliance on the First Amendment. The scope of the Amendment is subject to judicial interpretation and First Amendment rights are not absolute. Speech is not protected if defamatory or if it incites disruption, including disruption to office or business operations (*Connick v. Myers*, 461 US 138 150-51 (1983)).

Thus while some protection is given to whistleblowers at common law the scope of protection given by the courts is limited. A whistleblower may be in a better position if he can establish that his disclosure is protected by statute.

Statutory protection

A large number of statutes at both state and federal level protect whistleblowers. But their impact on health care employees is more limited than might at first appear. Many statutes simply protect one particular group of employees and are of no help in the context of health care. For example, one of the most famous whistleblowing statutes in the US is the Civil Service Reform Act 1978 which allows civil servants to disclose malpractice and wrongdoing and sets up federal organisations to investigate these complaints. However, the Act only covers employees of the federal civil service.

Certain general antidiscrimination statutes give some protection from retaliation to persons who blow the whistle on matters covered by the statute. Perhaps the most celebrated statute at federal level is the Title VII Civil Rights Act 1964. Title VII is an antiretaliation provision which makes it unlawful for an employer to take any reprisals against an employee who makes a complaint, testifies, assists or otherwise participates in an investigation concerning discrimination on the basis of race, colour, religion, sex and national origin. This protection is not automatic. For example, an employee's conduct may be 'so excessive and so deliberately calculated to inflict needless economic hardship on the employer' that it loses the protection of Title VII. (*EEOC v. Kallir Phillip Ross Inc.*, 401 F. Supp 66 71 (DC NY 1975) 10 EPD 10 366). Similar antidiscrimination statutes apply to the states. Various federal labour laws protect persons who have filed charges or given testimony under the Act. For example, the Fair Labor Standards Act protects all persons (not just employees) from retaliation and the Occupational Safety and Health Act 1976 deals with complaints to other agencies regarding regular workplace safety. There are difficulties, however, for whistleblowers seeking to rely on such general statutes because they are too broad to have a positive impact (Malin, 1987).

Even if whistleblowers can show that they are protected by an applicable statute they must show that their disclosure was sanctioned under the legislation. Private sector employees are less favoured by legislative protection than public sector employees. In New York private employees are protected when revealing *actual* violations of law (Labor Law 740). This legislation only covers certain disclosures, relating to violations of the law that present 'a substantial and specific danger to health and safety' (Labor Law S740(2)). Disclosures relating to white collar crimes such as fraud are excluded. In contrast the Civil Service Law (75-b) applies to public employees in New York City if they disclose information on what they reasonably believe to be improper government conduct.

Even if the information disclosed is within the category protected by statute this does not mean that an employee may voice his concerns to the world at large. Statutes usually specify the person/organisation to whom complaints should be made. While federal statutes encourage both internal and external whistleblowing, in contrast many state statutes require the whistleblower to disclose outside the institution (Morehead *et al.*, 1991). But this whistleblowing must be within defined channels. Whistleblowing to the media is often banned (Morehead *et al.*, 1991). It has been suggested that one reason for encouraging external whistleblowing is that it leads to improved investigations of such things as illegality or misconduct. However, internal whistleblowing has some advantages. It allows an organisation to react to the complaint and perhaps remedy the problem. Organisations may as a result become more responsive to complaints. But to simply rely on internal whistleblowing is likely to be insufficient. Requiring complaints to be made to one specified person gives that person considerable power to undermine the whistleblower.

Despite the veritable plethora of whistleblowing statutes it is noticeable how few claims have been brought under them. Moreover, even where actions have been brought, success is not guaranteed. A study published in 1987 revealed that over a four year period only three appellate cases in the three states studied concerned employees who had sought protection under the statutes and these employees had only limited success (Dworkin and Near, 1987). It was suggested that the reason for the failure of the statutes was the errors in legislative drafting and ineffective interpretation. A practical difficulty in bringing claims is the frequent delays in waiting for them to be processed. As Westin (1981) has commented, this means that:

> Many employees and executives face periods of waiting during which they may be fired from their job, cannot get good references and have no legal determination of validity of their complaint to offer to potential employers.

If the whistleblower's claim is upheld he may be awarded compensation. This may take the form of equitable damages which encompass reinstatement, back pay, restoration of seniority, fringe benefits and actual damages which include tort remedies available for wrongful dismissal, for example, non-economic damages for emotional distress. A few states allow punitive damages. It is unlikely, however, that reinstatement will be ordered since, as in the UK, this is a remedy which the courts are unwilling to use.

Perhaps the most important reason behind the unwillingness to disclose is that employees regard the personal cost of disclosure to be too heavy to pay. As Fisher (1991) comments:

> Whistleblowers are not team players. This is an era of team players. Hence the tension; people hate waste, fraud and corruption that whistleblowers expose but they also hate the whistleblowers who expose it and thereby refuse to be part of the team.

Even in the context of the federal civil service where perhaps some of the most comprehensive whistleblowing protection exists, whistleblowers are unwilling to come forward and disclose. A former Special Counsel (one of the officials appointed to investigate whistleblowers' complaints) has commented that:

> I'd say that unless you are in a position to retire or independently wealthy, don't do it. Don't put your head up because it will be blown off.
> (Fisher, 1991)

The whistleblowers may face opposition from workmates and others in bringing a claim. Steps may be taken against him, ranging from sending him to Siberia (the systematic freezing of the whistleblower from corporate life) through to rationalisation of jobs with the elimination of that of the whistleblower.

The small numbers of whistleblowers are a source of concern, so much so in fact that in some states whistleblowing incentives have been introduced. For example, in Oregon whistleblowers can collect up to $250 if this is an amount greater than would be the damages awarded in a suit based on retaliation for whistleblowing. In South Carolina the whistleblower may be awarded 25% of any savings resulting from whistleblowing in the first year up to a maximum of $2000. Financial compensation for whistleblowers has been allowed for many years in the federal False Claims Act which is designed to allow recovery of money taken falsely by government contractors. This allows for more substantial claims than the state statutes. The False Claims Act provides that if the government chooses to prosecute an action taken by a relator then the relator receives 15–25% of any treble damages and fines recovered from the defendant. To obtain a reward the wrongdoing must be brought to the attention of the government through a law suit being filed. Cumbersome procedure has led to recovery under the Act being delayed in some cases by a year or more. Fears of claims by unscrupulous persons have not, however, materialised, largely since without government assistance individuals are unlikely to proceed.

Making rewards available is unlikely dramatically to increase the incidence of whistleblowing. In many cases individuals blow the whistle because they are acting on the basis of conscience rather than personal gain. Rewards may actually deter disclosure by those who are motivated to disclose out of organisational loyalty. Research by sociologists has shown that those who are more likely to claim rewards are younger persons and individuals with low self-esteem. Morehead *et al.* (1992) suggest that before more legislation is introduced more information on the efficacy of awards needs to be obtained.

There has been renewed pressure for more federal legislation to safeguard whistleblowers. In 1988 Senator Howard Metzenbaum sponsored a Uniform Health and Safety Whistleblowers Protection Act. If enacted this would have protected any employee from retaliatory discharge for disclosing any activity, policy or practice by the employer that the employee reasonably believed to be a violation of any health and safety law. A bill was also introduced into Congress by Eugene Fiddell recommending that a single federal statute should be enacted recognising whistleblowing in health care; however, the bill died in committee.

One final point in relation to the United States which appears to be unclear is whether failure to blow the whistle could itself render a health care professional liable. In *Tarasoff v. Regents of the University of California* (529 p 22d 553 118 Cal R 14 (1976)) a court in California indicated that a duty was placed upon health care professionals to take reasonable steps to warn a person who was likely to be endangered by the action of another person if the health care professional became aware of this. This obligation to disclose outweighed the obligation to keep medical information confidential. It is unclear whether the courts in the United States would be prepared to impose such a duty upon a health care professional who saw malpractice or a poor standard of care and did not disclose his concern. There is no corresponding widespread duty of disclosure recognised in English law although some judicial statements indicate that such a duty does exist (*W v. Egdell* [1989] 1 All ER 1085).

Conclusions

Standards of health care provision may be scrutinised through a number of different mechanisms in the USA but none of these mechanisms has met with universal approval. Professionals may feel that the only way for grievances to be aired is to blow the whistle but while some recognition has been given to whistleblowers in law in the United States it is very limited in its extent. Nevertheless the US experience illustrates that whistleblowing may have significant repercussions. In Ms Bardenilla's case her medical treatment was investigated and doctors were charged with murder. While they were eventually acquitted, the case had a big impact on subsequent 'termination of treatment' cases in the United States (*Superior Court of the State of California for the County of Los Angeles-People of the State v. Neil Barber and Robert Negdi* (1983)).

Admittedly recognition of whistleblowing has its drawbacks. Not all whistleblowers are heroes or heroines (Howard, 1988). As Fisher (1991) comments, there is the danger that individuals may attempt to use whistleblowing as a means of insulating themselves from their own incompetence. Individuals who anticipate that they may be in line for dismissal could blow the whistle on malpractice and then claim that their eventual dismissal was due not to their own incompetence but to their whistleblowing.

In addition, as Winslow has commented in the context of nursing advocacy:

> Most of us acknowledge loyalty to associates as a virtue. An unwillingness to expose a colleague's shortcomings to public view and a desire to preserve confidence in one's institution are among the characteristic features of loyalty. Deeming such loyalty a vice would be a mistake likely to produce detrimental results for both health care providers and patients.
>
> (Winslow, 1984)

Whistleblowing should ideally be a last resort. It is far better for institutions to be responsive to claims of poor standards of care or allegations of malpractice and for them to have adequate internal mechanisms to receive complaints and to resolve problems. Perhaps the time has come in the United States, as in the UK, for a thorough overhaul of complaints procedures. But admittedly while this may be the ideal, in practice simple reliance upon internal disclosure is unlikely to be enough. Even the best designed complaints procedures may break down and those in positions of authority may choose to disregard complaints. Nevertheless, loyalty may have to give way at some point to broader issues of public policy. This may arise when standards of care are in danger. If the patient is at risk this needs to be made public.

Eugene Fiddell's initiative in advocating a federal statute for health care workers is to be welcomed but such a statute needs to be accompanied by a thorough re-examination of the other mechanisms for scrutiny of care which exist at both state and federal level.

Acknowledgements

The author would like to thank Linda Mulcahney, Eugene Fiddell, Timothy Jost, Anne McBride and Melanie Wilson Silver for their help. The author remains, of course, responsible for all opinions expressed and any errors which may remain.

References

ARON, M. (1992) Whistleblowers, Insubordination and Employee Rights of Free Speech. *Labor Law Journal*, 211–220.

BLUMBERG, P. (1971) Corporate Responsibility and the Employee's Duty of Loyalty and Obedience; A Preliminary Enquiry. *Oklahoma Law Review* **24(3)**, 279.

CAPRON, A. (1988) A national committee on medical ethics. In *Health Rights and Resources*, P. Byrne (ed.). Wiley, London.

CURRENT TOPICS (1989) New US Legislation in 1989 for the better protection of whistleblowers. *Australian Law Journal*, 592.

DWORKIN, T. M. AND NEAR, J. P. (1987) Whistleblowing statutes: are they working? *American Business Law Journal* **25**, 241.

FISHER, B. D. (1991) Whistleblower Protection Act 1989 – a false hope for whistleblowers. *Rutgers Law Review* **43**, 355–417.

FRIEDSON, E. (1987) *Medical Work in America*. Yale University Press, Connecticut.

FURROW, B. R. *et al.* (1981) *Health Law*, 2nd ed. West Publishing, St Paul, Minn.

FRY, S. (1989) Whistleblowing by nurses: a matter of ethics. *Nursing Outlook* 37(1), 56.

GIBSON, S. and KUSHER, H. (1986) Ethics committees. How are they doing? *Hastings Centre Report* 16, 975.

MYRON GLAZER (1983) Ten Whistleblowers and How They Fared. *Hastings Centre Report*, 33–41.

HAYNES, D. S. (1988) The current status of the doctrine of employment at will. *Labor Law Journal* 39(1), 19–32.

HOWARD, J. C. (1988) Current developments in whistleblower protection. *Labor Law Journal* 39(2), 67.

JOST, T., MULCAHY, L., STRASSER, S. AND SACHS, L. (1993) Consumer complaints and professional discipline. *Health Matrix*.

MALIN, M. H. (1983) Protecting the whistleblower from retaliatory discharge. *University of Michigan Journal of Law Reform* 16(2), 277–318.

McCALL SMITH, A. (1990) Committee ethics? Clinical ethics committees and their introduction in the United Kingdom. *Journal of Law and Society* 17(1), 124.

MICHAEL, J. (1981) *The Politics of Secrecy*. Penguin, Harmondsworth.

MORAN, M. AND WOOD, B. (1993) *States, Regulation and the Medical Profession*. Oxford University Press, Oxford.

MOREHEAD, T., DWORKIN, T. M. AND CALLAHAN, E. S. (1991) Internal whistleblowing protecting the interests of the employee, the organization and society. *American Business Law Journal* 29, 266–308.

MOREHEAD, T., DWORKIN, T. M. AND CALLAHAN, E. S. (1992) Do good and get rich; financial incentives for whistleblowers and the False Claims Act. *Villanova Law Review* 37, 273–336.

PETERSON, J. C. AND FARRELL, D. (1986) *Whistleblowing, ethical and legal issues in expressing dissent*. Kendall Hunt, Illinois, USA.

RAFFEL, M. W. (1989) *The U.S. Health System: Origins and Functions*. Delmar Publishers, New York.

RONGINE, N. M. (1985) Towards a coherent legal response to the public policy dilemma posed by whistleblowing. *American Business Law Journal* 23, 281–97.

ROSENTHALL, M. (1988) *Dealing with Medical Malpractice*. Tavistock Publishing, London.

ROSENTHALL, M. (1992) Medical discipline in cross-cultural perspective; the United States, Britain and Sweden. In *Quality and Regulation in Health Care*, R. Dingwall and P. Fenn (eds). Routledge, London.

STEINBOCK, B. (1983) The removal of Herbert's feeding tube. *Hastings Centre Report* **13**, 13–16.

WESTIN, A. (1981) *Whistleblowing*. McGraw Hill, New York.

WINSLOW, G. (1984) From loyalty to advocacy: a new metaphor for nursing. *Hastings Centre Report* **14**(3), 32–40.

10

Two initiatives to reform accountability

Jean McHale

Two responses to the growing public debate surrounding whistleblowing deserve special attention – one from the Conservative Government and one from an opposition MP. In October 1992 the Department of Health circulated for consultation draft guidance on freedom of speech in the NHS. The following month a Bill was introduced by Derek Fatchett MP (Labour), namely the National Health Service (Freedom of Speech) Bill 1992. The Department of Health's *Guidance for Staff on Relations with the Public and the Media* was published in June 1993 (DoH, 1993). This chapter seeks to examine how far these initiatives have advanced the whistleblowing debate and to what extent further reform is still required (see also McHale, 1992, 1993a).

The government guidance

The *Guidance* begins by stating that individual NHS staff have both a right and a duty to raise with their employer any matter of concern about health service issues concerned with the delivery of care or services to the patient or client. The recognition of the need of employees to speak out here is to be welcomed. However, the exact meaning of a duty to disclose is unclear. What would the consequences be for employees who did not disclose? Will they be subject to disciplinary action? There is no obligation at present recognised in English law upon a health care professional to disclose information where this may cause harm to another person. Such a duty has been recognised in the United States in the case of *Tarasoff v. Regents of the University of California* (California Reports 129 529p 2nd 553 (1974)). It is uncertain at present if English law would impose such a duty to disclose information upon a health care professional. There has been some judicial support for a duty to disclose where the public may be at risk in the case of *W v. Egdell* ([1989] 1 All ER 1085). Were such a duty to be recognised in English law this might have a considerable impact upon the scope of medical confidentiality if health care professionals feel obliged to disclose information to avoid becoming liable in the law of tort (McHale, 1989).

The second principle in the *Guidance* is that NHS employers should ensure that local policies and procedures are introduced to allow these rights and duties to be fully and properly met. It is emphasised that there must be adequate internal procedures for resolving disputes. In an ideal world organisations should have a level of openness such that employees are willing to vent their concerns and employers are sufficiently responsive to those expressed concerns.

The government emphasises that first, complaints should be made informally between an individual and his immediate line manager. But, as has been pointed out by many of the organisations which responded during the consultation period of the draft *Guidance*, this may not be the most appropriate method of complaint. Many of the complaints may relate to how low to middle management implement policies or operate their units. As the legal advice centre Public Concern at Work commented:

> To require a concerned member of staff to confront his or her line manager on their judgement or priorities in this way is unlikely to be productive or conducive for a good working environment. Only the most exceptional manager would not, in such a situation, want to pull rank over the staff member concerned.

Karen Jennings of the union COHSE (now UNISON) said, before the *Guidance* was issued, 'In a sense, to complain direct to the line manager is to cook your own goose' (*The Times*, 1992).

The *Guidance* distinguishes between those health care professionals who are in a direct line management relationship and others such as consultants who are not in such a relationship. Concerning the latter it is suggested that they discuss their concerns with relevant colleagues and then take the matter up directly with the general manager or chief executive. This difference in approach between NHS employees may be seen as undesirable and indeed as divisive.

There is a further problem with using informal procedures for voicing concerns since, as Brown and McKenna (1992) comment, if employees make an informal complaint they may have no proof of having made the complaint. This may prejudice them at any subsequent disciplinary proceedings. The *Guidance* recommends that formal procedures be established for the situation in which an informal approach appears to be ineffective. The formal procedure should allow complaints to be referred up the management line.

The *Guidance* provides (Clause 18) that it should be made clear to an employee whether they could be accompanied or represented by their professional organisation or trade union representative or a person of their choice. It is submitted that this suggestion does not go far enough and that there should be an automatic right to representation. The guidelines provide that ultimately an employee should be able to go to the highest level of local management and finally to the chair of the health authority or trust. The highest level of appeal is within the existing management framework. There is no external right of appeal within the *Guidance*. This, it is submitted, is unsatisfactory. If matters of public policy are involved here it surely requires some external input.

An alternative approach to using all the levels of the management chain, which the *Guidance* proposes (Clause 21), may be for a designated officer to be given the role of receiving complaints. This is to be a senior officer and it may be the officer who is designated to receive patients' complaints under the complaints procedure established by the Hospital Complaints Act 1985. But the designated officer under this Act is frequently the unit general manager and they may not be the most appropriate person to perform this role. First, they are part of the line management and a health care professional may feel inhibited in approaching them because of a lack of perceived independence. Second, there is a danger that the unit general manager may not have adequate time to devote to the consideration of staff complaints since they have many tasks to undertake. It has been suggested by the whistleblowers' network Freedom to Care that they be required to compile reports on the number and nature of concerns raised and the designated officer action taken. This would enable complaints to be monitored and action taken over poor standards to be co-ordinated at a higher level.

The *Guidance* suggests that if complaints are made to a designated officer and the matter is not resolved then the issue should be referred to the chair of the authority or trust for action to be taken.

Confidentiality

Another potential difficulty caused by the *Guidance* is the approach taken to the question of maintaining the confidentiality of patient information. Health care professionals are required by their ethical codes to maintain patient confidentiality and this stipulation is also often contained in their contracts of employment. However, there may be occasions when to show that standards of care have fallen, it may be necessary to reveal details of individual cases. In such a situation the health care professional is torn between an obligation of confidentiality and the public interest in ensuring the health of patients and the need to uphold good standards of patient care.

This tension was shown in the case of nurse Graham Pink (Pink, 1992). The relatives of an elderly patient whose case was referred to by Mr Pink in his disclosures claimed that they could recognise their relative from the description given in the newspaper (although no names had been used). Mr Pink was disciplined on grounds of breach of confidence. While he was required to keep patient confidentiality his ethical code also required him to take note of unsatisfactory standards of care (UKCC, 1992, secs. 11–13).

The *Guidance* does not assist the health care professional in resolving this conflict. It refers to the duty of confidentiality to preserve patient information and the duty of confidentiality and loyalty to the employer (Clauses 8, 9). Should employees break these duties they would find themselves subject to disciplinary action. It recognises, however, that this duty of confidence is not absolute. In law if an authorised disclosure of confidential medical information is made the remedy of breach of confidence may be used to restrain disclosure (*X v. Y* [1988] QB 68). But an action for breach of confidence will not succeed if the disclosure is made in the public interest (see Ch. 11). In *Gartside v. Outram*, Wood said 'There is no confidence in the disclosure of iniquity' ((1857) 26 LJ Ch (NS) 113). The courts have interpreted iniquity as something which goes beyond such things as disclosure of information relating to a crime. In *Beloff v. Pressdram* Thomas said that 'disclosure of information where it relates to matters medically dangerous to the public' is justified (1 All ER 241). It is submitted that the public have an interest in the disclosure of information relating to falling standards of health care.

But while there may be a public interest in some disclosure that does not mean that the public interest requires that information be disclosed to the public as a whole. In *Initial Services v. Putterill* Lord Denning held that disclosure would only be allowed where it was made to a person with a proper interest in receiving the information ([1976] 3 All ER 145). In *Attorney General v. Guardian Newspapers* the court held that disclosure of information concerning the security services only amounted to disclosure in the public interest where this disclosure was made to the proper authorities ((1988) 3 WLR 776). But in some situations general disclosure is not in the public interest. In *Lion Laboratories v. Evans* the court held that disclosure to the press of defects in a breathalyser machine was justifiable ([1984] 2 All ER 47).

The *Guidance* provides that since the decision to disclose in the public interest may well be challenged, the employee would be well advised to seek advice from a specialist advice agency.

It has been suggested by Freedom to Care in their response to the *Guidance* that one compromise over the problem of breach of confidence would be to allow disclosures to be made but without identifying names. While this is a helpful suggestion it is submitted that it is not sufficient. The *Guidance* does not address the problem of a sliding scale of confidentiality within the NHS (McHale, 1993b, Ch. 4). Information concerning certain medical conditions is by its very nature sensitive, for example, relating to the treatment of patients who have developed

AIDS or venereal disease. Other medical conditions are generally unlikely to be seen as being of such an inherently confidential nature, such as a broken arm. The *Guidance* does not begin to address these complexities.

The *Guidance*, moreover, does not take account of the fact that information differs between that relating to medical conditions and other types of information, for example, commercially sensitive information. A major review of the confidentiality of patient information within the NHS is being undertaken by the government and it is to be hoped that this will provide clarification of the boundaries of disclosure.

Outside agencies

The *Guidance* makes reference to the fact that in some situations health care professionals may wish to consult with outside agencies. For example, Clause 27 refers to the Mental Health Act Commission; where an NHS employee is concerned about the welfare of a patient detained under the Mental Health Act 1983 he may decide to take his complaint to the Commission.

Clause 26 refers to the Health Service Commissioner (the Ombudsman). Issues similar to those which concerned Mr Pink have been investigated by the Health Service Commissioner. One of the largest categories of complaint the Commissioner has been concerned with involves the management of elderly and handicapped patients. The Commissioner has already indicated that he is willing to receive complaints from hospital staff on behalf of patients (HMSO, 1992a). However, there are difficulties in reliance on the Commissioner some of which were noted by the Patients' Association in their written response to the draft *Guidance*. The Commissioner's office has very limited resources and it may take a long time to process a claim. In addition the Commissioner is restricted in the matters to which he can refer. At present the Commissioner can examine complaints that a failure in the health service or maladministration has resulted in injustice or hardship. He can review the operation of a number of health service bodies such as hospitals, ambulance services and district nursing services. However, certain areas are removed from his scrutiny; for example, he cannot consider complaints concerning general practitioners and is unable to investigate complaints relating to matters of clinical judgement. However if a medical practitioner claims that a certain issue is a matter of clinical judgement and thus outside the Commissioner's jurisdiction, the Commissioner may still decide to review that claim. Where a complaint is made and is found to be justified he may recommend that the Department of Health make changes in clinical practice.

The *Guidance* makes explicit reference (Clause 23) to the fact that all staff have a right to consult a professional agency such as a trade union or other representative agencies. It also suggests (Clause 27) that when all other mechanisms of complaint have been exhausted the employee might wish to consult his MP in confidence or go to the media but if such action was taken unjustifiably disciplinary action could be taken. This clause came under considerable criticism with MPs protesting at the threat to health care professionals who wanted to exercise their constitutional right of access to an MP. Following the storm of criticism in November 1993 Sir Duncan Nichol issued a statement to say that the government had not intended to interfere with the constitutional right of access to an MP and that the clause concerning disciplinary proceedings was intended simply to refer to disclosures to the media (BMJ, 1993).

Blowing the whistle to the press

In view of the fact that the guidelines are entitled *Guidance to NHS Staff on Relations with the Public and the Media* it is perhaps ironic that it is only at the very end of the guidelines that the question of the media is addressed (Clause 28):

> Such action (disclosure to the media) if entered into unjustifiably could result in disciplinary action and might unreasonably undermine public confidence in the Service.
> In view of these considerations any employee contemplating making a disclosure to the media is advised to first seek further specialist guidance from professional and other representative bodies and to discuss matters further with his or her colleagues and, where appropriate line and professional managers. In the light of the principles set out in this guidance however and the fact that local procedures will have been determined in consultation with local staff and staff representatives, it is expected that proper mechanisms will exist to ensure that staff concerns can be addressed and dealt with without reference to the media.

This paragraph makes it quite plain that disclosure to the media is to be a matter of last resort with staff being careful of the consequences. However, it does not refer to the fact that disclosure to the press may be held to be justifiable where it is in the public interest. The *Guidance* cannot, of course, address the general failure to protect whistleblowers in English law. There is no general statutory protection for whistleblowers, nor is there any specific statutory protection for whistleblowers in health care.

The Fatchett Bill

In late 1992 Derek Fatchett MP introduced a Bill with the aim of providing increased openness in the NHS: the *National Health Service (Freedom of Speech) Bill*. The Bill did not find sufficient support in Parliament but is a useful basis for discussion of reform here.

The Bill began by attempting to impose a general ethical code on all health care employees. Many NHS employees are already subject to an ethical code drawn up by their respective professional body such as the GMC or the UKCC (UKCC, 1992; GMC, 1993). There has also been discussion as to whether NHS managers should be concerned with ethics (Wall, 1989). This is particularly important in view of the many resource allocation decisions which they are called upon to make. The Fatchett Bill recommended that a 'charter of values' be drawn up in relation to NHS staff, a task to be undertaken by the Secretary of State, having regard to existing ethical codes of conduct of health professionals. While it is important to ensure that ethical considerations are taken into account, is the introduction of yet another ethical code the solution? Health care professionals within the NHS may find themselves obligated by their contract of employment to follow one ethical code and by their professional body to follow another. This may be a recipe for confusion. A further problem posed by this recommendation relates to the fact that the Fatchett Bill applies only to NHS employees. Professionals in private health care would presumably continue to be governed by their original ethical code.

The Bill does not specify the content of the ethical code in detail. However, it did provide that the charter should include:

> a duty and a right to report to any competent person any instruction, policy or practice which they believe would result in inadequate or unsafe conditions which are likely to either harm the health, safety or well-being of patients/clients or colleagues or be contrary to law or be to the detriment of the health service and public confidence in its operation.
>
> (Fatchett, 1992)

The difficulty with this type of obligation is that it could give rise to problems of interpretation in the same way as the nurses' ethical code presents such problems. The Bill left open the question of who was the competent person to whom disclosure had to be made. Is this simply a member of line management? Furthermore, as with the *Guidance*, while the Fatchett Bill provided that there should be a duty to disclose it is not stated as to what the consequences will be should a health care professional not disclose. Would the courts be prepared to extend the law of tort to require that health care professionals are under a duty to disclose where the public interest is at risk?

The legislative proposals made by Fatchett provided (Clause 8) that model 'concern procedures' should be drawn up. These would allow NHS staff to express their concerns regarding poor standards of care at local level. Procedures were to be drawn up after full consultation with interested persons and organisations including trade unions and professional bodies representing NHS staff. Formal procedures were to be instituted for the identification, reporting and investigation of staff concerns. Investigations should be undertaken by an appropriate manager or by another person designated by the employing authority. There should be time limits placed upon investigation of these concerns. Written notification of the outcome of an investigation should be made to the staff member who had made the complaint. In addition there should be a right of appeal to a panel of the employing authority.

The Fatchett Bill does not make the scope of these procedures clear. We are not told who is to be given the task of handling complaints. It is likely that Fatchett was here referring to managerial resolution of complaints since he separates from this investigating provision a right of external appeal to an investigating body. This recommendation, if enacted, would have led to much the same problems as are presented by the *Guidance* if reliance is placed upon line management to perform this role. Where the Bill differs from the *Guidance* is in the inclusion of a right of external appeal. This right of external appeal should apply in two situations. First, where the internal appeal structure had been exhausted an appeal would be made as to a higher body. Second, a staff member should be able to go to the tribunal where there was an immediate or urgent threat to the safety, health or well-being of patients or of the employee's colleagues. This would provide a useful means for complaints to be discussed without the issue being aired totally in public – a form of controlled disclosure. The involvement of an external body would enhance perceived independence. The Bill provides that the new appeal body would be appointed by the Secretary of State. She would have the task of ensuring that the body was independent and was qualified to undertake its tasks. The Secretary of State should consult with interested persons or organisations. In determining what body should take on the role she should consider the role to be played by community health councils and by the Health Service Commissioner.

There is at present no obvious candidate for the role of external appeal body. Would community health councils or the Health Service Commissioner be an appropriate body? Community health councils are bodies composed of members nominated by the local authority, local voluntary organisations and by the regional health authority (see Ch. 5). They have a duty to represent the interests of the public in their health district and, where it is proposed to make a substantial variation or a substantial development in health services, they must be consulted (DoH, 1985). The councils face difficulties in performing their existing role. It appears that the information which they receive is frequently inadequate to enable them to make full comment (Longley, 1990). Moreover the members of the council are not fulltime appointments and this limits their ability to deal with cases. The councils as presently constituted would not be suitable to perform the role of an appeal body. Radical reform would be required. Perhaps the most fundamental objection to the use of community health councils here is that they operate on a regional basis whereas it would be more appropriate for such a body to be national.

One alternative is for the Health Service Commissioner's office to be expanded. But would this be suitable? The scope of his investigating powers would have to be reviewed. His office would require more resources. While the Commissioner has already made recommendations with implications for management practice, to give him a broader role would necessarily involve him still further in the decisions of management.

It would also surely be insufficient for an external agency to simply act as a source of appeal. It is vital to ensure that there is a more general scrutiny of health care standards. Firefighting when things go wrong is all very well but it is far better to institute an effective system of firewatching. An external agency should, it is suggested, perform both roles. Its role would surely need to be linked to a more general overview of the standards of health care. In their recommendations on whistleblowing issued before the *Guidance*, the Royal College of Nursing suggested that the government should set an agreed standard of care for each health care service using an objective standard setting procedure (RCN, 1992). A further recommendation was that a national inspectorate for health care be established along the lines of the original inspectorate for education. This is the path down which clinical practice is moving. Medical audit has been introduced on a national basis. Would this not surely be the next logical step? The Bill provided that the independent agency should investigate issues referred to it. If the investigation revealed matters of general application they should be brought to the attention of NHS managers and staff and of interested organisations such as trade unions and professional bodies. The body was also to have the role of ensuring that staff who raise concerns in good faith are not subject to penalty, detriment or disciplinary action. Doubts may be cast by some on the powers of reporting back contained in the bill. Should this really include reporting back to a trade union? Some might argue that this is tantamount to general public disclosure.

The Bill recommends that the independent body should ensure that the NHS employee is not subject to penalty but fails to state just how this praiseworthy suggestion is to be achieved. Ensuring that discrimination did not take place would be an exceedingly difficult task. Would this need separate legislation? Even if such legislative machinery were instituted there would still be the problem that whistleblowers have never been fully accepted. Even in the United States where whistle-blowing in the civil service has been long recognised, there is still unwillingness to recognise the whistleblower (see Ch. 9).

A blueprint for reform or the source of fresh controversy?

Both the Fatchett Bill and the government's *Guidance* fail to consider the advocacy movement. The main thrust of advocacy has come in recent years from the nursing profession. One model of this is the nurse acting as an advocate for her patient by advancing her patient's rights; for example, the nurse voicing her concern that the treatment being given is not appropriate for that patient or that a patient is being given insufficient information regarding treatment. More recently, advocacy has become nationally recognised. Some areas of health care have been particularly concerned with the development of the advocacy movement, such as the care of the mentally ill. The Ashworth Inquiry into abuses at Ashworth special hospital included in their recommendations support for a funded system of patient advocates (HMSO, 1992b). The advocacy movement has led to the development of patient representatives, individuals expressly appointed to act on behalf of patients within individual hospitals. A research project was established by the National Association of Hospitals and by the King's Fund Centre and in 1993 a patient repre-sentative forum was set up with approximately 25 members.

The failure of both the Fatchett and government initiatives to deal with the issue of the professional as advocate is surely a considerable omission. If health care professionals are acting as advocates then they are more likely to regard their foremost duty as being owed to the patient. This would surely have a considerable impact on decisions to disclose to the public.

A further failure of both the *Guidance* and the Fatchett Bill is that they do not address the overlap between staff complaints and patient complaints procedures. The latter were established under the Hospital Complaints Act 1985. It is surely illogical to have two separate systems operating alongside each other. The government has recently indicated that it is considering introducing conciliators into hospitals (Times, 1994) but rather than simply taking remedial measures for diffusing concern, more thorough reform is required. In the United States hospitals have complaints mechanisms and some hospitals have appointed patient representatives or patient ombudsmen who can receive complaints from staff or patients (see Ch. 9). National co-ordination of patient representatives is required as part of a general complaints structure. Having an independent person within a hospital may make employees more willing to come forward and less fearful for the consequences for their careers.

Both the Fatchett Bill and the *Guidance* concern complaints within the NHS but do not extend to cover private medicine. If whistleblowing by staff is seen as a matter of the management of a particular organisation then it is appropriate to let the organisation itself resolve the problem. However, if whistleblowing is seen as a wider social issue and a method of ensuring accountability then reforms should apply in the voluntary and private sectors too. This is particularly important in view of the fact that through the new contracting arrangements in the NHS, the care of NHS patients may be entrusted to non-NHS providers (Brazier, 1993, p. 193).

Conclusion

The whistleblowing debate looks set to continue. In an increasingly consumer driven society, surely it is right that health care providers both public and private should be accountable for the service provided and that deficiencies in care should be identified, whether by those within or outside the organisation. A more radical examination of the procedures in existence for the scrutiny of private and NHS care is required than anything which has been attempted up to now.

References

BMJ (1993) Whistleblowers may tell MPs. *British Medical Journal* **307**, 1216.

BRAZIER, M. (1993) *Medicine, Patients and the Law*. Penguin, Harmondsworth.

BROWN, D. AND McKENNA, B. (1992) NHS workers: whistling in the dark. *Solicitors Journal* **136**, 994.

DoH (1985) *Community Health Council Regulations*, S.I. No. 304 reg. 18. HMSO, London.

DoH (1993) *Guidance for Staff on Relations with the Public and Media*. DoH, London.

FATCHETT D. (1992) National Health Service (Freedom of Speech) Bill Ordered by Manufacturing, Science, Finance to be printed, 10th December 1992, London.

GMC (1993) *Professional Conduct and Fitness to Practise (Blue Book)*. GMC, London.

HMSO (1992a) *Health Service Commissioner's Annual Report for 1991–92*, HC82. HMSO, London.

HMSO (1992b) *Report of the Committee of Inquiry into Complaints at Ashworth Special Hospital*. HMSO, London.

LONGLEY, D. (1990) Diagnostic dilemmas: accountability in the NHS. *Public Law*, 527–52.

MCHALE, J. (1989) Confidentiality: an absolute obligation'. Modern Law Review **52**(5), 715–21.

MCHALE, J. (1992) Whistleblowing in the NHS. *Journal of Social Welfare & Family Law* **5**, 363–71.

MCHALE, J. (1993a) Whistleblowing in the NHS Revisited. *Journal of Social Welfare & Family Law* **1**, 52–7.

MCHALE, J. (1993b) *Medical Confidentiality and Legal Privilege*. Routledge, London.

PINK, G. (1992) *Truth from the Bedside*. Charter 88, London.

RCN (1992) *Whistleblow: Nurses Speak Out*. RCN, London.

THE TIMES (1992) Report, 7th August.

THE TIMES (1994) Report, 3rd January.

UKCC (1992) *Code of Professional Conduct*. UKCC, London.

WALL, A. (1989) *Ethics and the Health Service Manager*. King Edward's Hospital Fund for London, London.

11

Confidentiality and the public interest

Alan Hannah

The substitution in the general use of the words 'master and servant' with 'employer and employee' since the 1950s is a reflection of the change in the public perception of the status of an employee. Statutory interference in, or regulation of, the previously almost unfettered contractual power of the master now ensures that an employee ought not to be dismissed at the whim of an employer (at least after the first two years of employment). The many other rights ancillary to the employment relationship are also now much more closely regulated by law, e.g. outlawing deductions from wages, sex and race discrimination. Restraint of trade clauses (which have always been construed as contrary to public policy) are nowadays scrutinised by the court more closely and more readily found to be unreasonable and unenforceable save only just enough to protect the legitimate interests of the employer.

In the tough commercial and industrial employment market one can more readily accept that an employer whose business survival depends on slim profit margins in a hotly competitive trading market needs to have the protection of the law in injuncting those employees who might seek to further their private interests unfairly at the expense of the corporate concern they abandoned. I am referring to the commercially valuable secrets or confidential information that they acquire during the course of their employment. Nowadays it is not simply a risk of a disgruntled or ambitious employee using the confidential information as a passport to other employment. Not infrequently those employees set up business in competition with the former employer.

Confidential information

There are generally recognised to be three categories or grades of information in commercial concerns:

1. information so easily available to the public that an employee can impart it or use it during and after employment;

2. confidential information which should not be disclosed during employment without breaching an implied duty to the employer to keep it confidential;
3. specific trade secrets which the employee is not entitled to use during and after employment.

For the legitimate protection of the employer's business an employer can expressly provide measures to reduce the risk of confidential information in (2) and (3) above being imparted; for example, preventing an employee from working for a competitor in a defined area for a certain period for the reasonable protection of the employer's business or preventing an employee from employing any of the staff of the former employer. So one can readily understand the commercial necessity for the protection of an employer. But what of the public sector?

Confidentiality in the NHS

I think it important to try to identify the different categories of information which are confidential in the NHS or statutory trust bodies acting within or outside the NHS.

First, there is the classically confidential information relating to patients whom the NHS is there to serve. This will include sensitive information imparted by the patient, about him or herself or members of the family and, depending on the circumstances, the nature of the ailment. The rationale of protecting and preserving this confidential information is serving the public interest in respecting the private wishes of patients/clients for their and their families' details to remain undisclosed save for 'a need to know basis' in the course of treatment and that a patient has confidence that the sensitive information imparted will remain undisclosed.

Secondly, we look at other information which the health authorities and their subordinate managers label or deem confidential. This will include financial information relating to resources and prices in the current competitive income generation activities within the NHS. Matters concerned with the personal lives of the staff in their personnel records and disciplinary matters are all areas which are legitimately confidential. How much of the information within the NHS is in fact rightly deemed or labelled confidential is a question which I address. Financial deficits, staffing levels, performance failures and successes, efficiency and the like would seem to me to be information which could embarrass health authority managers but in a public body serving the public and accountable to the public, I very much doubt if there are any legitimate grounds for the cover and secrecy so prevalent.

Exhausting internal remedies

Let us assume an NHS employee has a concern about a matter of public importance in his employing authority. It would not, in my view, be politically or strategically desirable for them to voice their concern publicly without first giving the health authority the opportunity of assessing whether or not they agree that there is a problem and if so, the opportunity of addressing and remedying it. There are a number of reasons for this: first, loyalty to the employer and second, if the remedy is in the gift of the employer it would seem to be common sense for the employer to have the opportunity to remedy without the glare of publicity. This therefore gives rise to an emphasis on self-regulation.

There should, therefore, in every health authority be a formal procedure for dealing with voiced concerns. The procedure should recognise and reflect a corporate intention to air such concerns and evaluate them within a recognised corporate code of ethics. There should be a clearly defined code of ethics which set out, as far as possible, the standards of performance and service. Shortcomings should be able to be reasonably easily identified against the code. There should be a well-defined, uncomplicated and effective procedure for dealing with complaints or concern. All relevant staff at senior level should be involved with the right of the complainant to appeal by way of review to the top level of management.

Deficiencies of self-regulation

Without detracting from the importance of the principle of self-regulation and the necessity of these procedures, I am mindful of their deficiencies. These include a natural unwillingness for the architects of any problem to recognise it, for that is tantamount to an admission of incompetence either in letting it occur or failing to recognise it before the potential whistleblower does, and the fact that the remedy might involve a conflict of interest.

What a whistleblower perceives as a problem might not be recognised as such by his colleagues. Blunted by coping for years with inadequate resources, the senior manager may find it anathema for an untainted young idealist to tell those so much wiser and more experienced what is wrong. For these reasons, colleagues might well stick together against the 'troublemaker' and, recognising that this is not a perfect world, adjudge that there is no problem.

Worst of all, there may be a cover-up to hide the problem, conceal the evidence or dispose of it and bundle out the complainant by promotion or dismissal.

There may be some issues of concern too serious to be dealt with by internal procedures. Criminal offences involving the public, the patients or public monies might, depending on the circumstances of each case and after being reported to management, be taken outside the employing authority to be dealt with by the appropriate agency, e.g. the police.

No satisfaction after exhausting internal procedures

So the conscientious employee, not yet a whistleblower, has exhausted the internal review framework. If their anxiety is recognised and well-founded and remedy follows, all well and good. But in many cases this will not occur. What then? At this stage I postulate the following possibilities:

1. The concern is not well-founded and what the complainant perceived as a problem is not so.
2. The complaint is well-founded but no remedy follows, perhaps for reasons of insufficient resources or an unwillingness to solve the problem by dismissing the perpetrators of it, or perhaps because of a 'lack of evidence'.
3. The complaint had some substance, but in the opinion of the authority the complainant has incorrectly perceived the gravity of the concern and in all the circumstances remedy is unnecessary.

The problem with each of these possibilities is that their outcome is a value judgement of the employer who is not only a defendant but also a judge in its own cause. Internal enquiries following serious incidents have usually been conducted out of the public gaze and rarely carry any weight outside the health authority. My own experience of these private internal enquiries, after assessing their worth against the weight of evidence and conclusions of a following public enquiry, is that they have been woefully investigated, are unobjective, self-interested and are more likely to administer a rap on the knuckles than sanction the dismissal of the wrongdoer.

In cases of serious crimes which should be reported to the police, it becomes a matter of concern if senior management is notified of the offence but nothing appears to be done about it.

Moral considerations of whistleblowing

An NHS employee, having exhausted the internal procedures available and being no further forward, considers their position. 'To blow or not to blow', that is the question. The whistleblower has to take on the risk that they are right in their complaint. Their subjective assessment will not help them if objectively the perception of the problem was wrong. The historically popular lawyers' 'reasonable man' test hypothesizes what the archetypal, fictitious, modern day, reasonable person would do or say. The dilemma facing a potential whistleblower has the elements of one or more of the following moral considerations:

1. To remedy by exposure a state of affairs in the interests of the public, which would otherwise continue to the detriment of the public. It would seem to be morally right to do so.
2. Courage. Any such action could bring the employee into disrepute with the employer.
3. Unselfishness. The employee who risks personal security and income for the public welfare can only be commended. If they lose their job, they seriously affect their own future employment 'marketability'.
4. The risk of injunctive relief and a claim for costs (horrific sums nowadays).

As to motive, if the principal purpose is revenge or financial gain, does it affect the morality of the exposure? If financial reward is a consequence, does the public interest absolve the moral turpitude, if any? These are philosophical questions which I shall answer only by illustrating the end parameters of the spectrum.

At the high moral end I place the whistleblower who risks their job (and future employment marketability) in exposing a state of affairs the continuation of which is contrary to the public interest. At the low moral end I picture the whistleblower who discovers a state of affairs and seeks as a principal and paramount objective financial gain by selling the story to a newspaper. As far as the public is concerned, in both these examples the result is the same and what ought to be exposed in the public good is so exposed.

Is the employee who does nothing to expose the wrong they discover because they either lack courage and/or decline for moral considerations to profit from the discovery worse or better than the exposer who for selfish reasons acts with the consequence of greater good for the public.

As I shall show later in this chapter, as far as legal considerations are concerned, it appears that motive (or malice) is irrelevant in considering public interest defences.

The extent of the publication

If the whistleblower has exhausted the internal procedures and potential remedies available (even perhaps by going to the Secretary of State) but without satisfaction, they will no doubt look for the next most effective step in redressing the perceived wrong. This is likely to involve publication in the sense that communication to anyone outside the health authority is in fact the public. At present there is no quango, commission, committee or ombudsman to whom special reference can be made.

A whistleblower is well advised to act reasonably at all relevant times and thus should look to the extent of the publication to ensure they do not overpublish. In most cases the most effective step is to involve the media of television and the press. Conceivably they could confine publication of, for example, financial irregularity and impropriety to the outside auditors of the employing health authority (even if they are auditors from a neighbouring health authority) to keep it out of the public eye. As far as the reasonableness of the actions is concerned (and I am contemplating the issues in an industrial tribunal hearing), I suggest that employees act reasonably if they confine publication to the appropriate body or, if there is no appropriate body, one could hardly criticise them if they go to the press. If the information is of sufficient public concern for an editor to publish it, then given the premise that the information is correct, the whistleblower is to some extent vindicated by the fact of publication.

Thus if they act reasonably in the extent of the publication and take the matter no further than is reasonably necessary at each appropriate stage but are still dismissed by the health authority, I suggest that they are less likely to have any compensation reduced by an industrial tribunal because of their own contribution to the dismissal (a power given to a tribunal in section 74(6) of the Employment Protection (Consolidation) Act 1978) should the dismissal eventually be found to be unfair.

Is motive irrelevant?

Motive may well be something to take into account in an industrial tribunal hearing, depending on the facts and the circumstances. But it is irrelevant to the issues of whether or not an injunction should be granted to prevent publication. Motive is generally speaking irrelevant as far as the courts are concerned (an exception being in defamation actions) as the courts are more concerned with the act and the particular intentions to do the act and not the reasons or motive for it.

In the case of *In re A Company's Application* ([1989] 3 WLR 265) the plaintiff company carried on business in the supply of financial advice and was regulated by FIMBRA pursuant to the Financial Services Act 1986. The defendant was a fairly senior employee who was dismissed but it was agreed he would continue with the plaintiff on a self-employed basis. Shortly after his dismissal he spoke to a senior executive of the plaintiff claiming damages, suggesting he would make confidential and embarrassing disclosures to FIMBRA unless his damages were paid. The plaintiff sought an injunction. It was held it would be contrary to public policy to forbid employees making appropriate confidential disclosures to a relevant statutory regulatory body and his motive for threatening those exposures was irrelevant.

What might be done

I do not believe the whistleblower in the NHS has materially much to gain if he exposes a scandal within the organisation in which he is employed. If the vested interests of the managers outweigh their perception of the public interest with the consequence of a dismissal, such dismissal is likely to be expressed on the grounds of a breach of confidentiality or breach of the term of mutual trust and confidence or some other reason embraced in the concept 'conduct' in section 57(2)(b) of the Employment Protection (Consolidation) Act 1978. A dismissal with perhaps more imagination on the part of the managers might be on the grounds of a (manufactured) redundancy. Even so, a hearing in the industrial tribunal, even if wholly successful on the part of the dismissed employee, still attracts only a maximum compensatory award of £11 000 together with a basic award equating to a redundancy payment.

The power given to an industrial tribunal to re-engage or reinstate is infrequently exercised and the fact that it is discretionary and not a right is small comfort for a whistleblower who, in the public interest, loses all. The courts (as opposed to the industrial tribunals) are unlikely to be of much assistance as they presently deal only with wrongful dismissals, i.e. dismissals resulting from a breach of contract.

A charter and an ombudsman?

Perhaps there should be an independent body, in the nature of an ombudsman-type committee, which operates by and under the principles expressed in a charter incorporating agreed guidelines for the raising of matters of public interest within the National Health Service. This committee might be charged with the task of investigating a complaint when the dismissed or career disadvantaged employee alone applies for a reference. I envisage the committee making its findings and recommendations after hearing both sides, adopting an inquisitorial procedure with no costs involved and no legal representation.

I entertain doubts whether such an independent body should be vested with any statutory power other than to make findings and recommendations, but perhaps industrial tribunals could (by way of an amendment to section 57 of the Employment Protection (Consolidation) Act 1978) be required to have due regard to those findings and recommendations in determining whether the dismissal was fair or unfair. If in the opinion of the industrial tribunal the employee was dismissed for raising matters of public concern and provided that employee acted substantially within the guidelines, and if the industrial tribunal finds the dismissal offended the spirit of the charter, perhaps it might be empowered to award up to double the maximum level of compensation, apart from its existing remedies as to reinstatement and re-engagement, and to award costs to the applicant.

Normally the industrial tribunal has jurisdiction to entertain a claim for unfair dismissal only after the employment has lasted two years. I think this period, in whistleblowing cases, should be reduced to nil, as in the case of dismissals of employees for trade union activities.

A policing role?

Let us briefly examine the responsibility of the health authority who, armed with highly confidential information from a patient, could save or protect the life of a member of the public by a breach of that confidential information. The various enquiries that have been held in child abuse and child death cases have now established the clear principle that a child's interests are paramount and that communication of confidential information on a 'need to know' basis only, and to the relevant agencies only, is justified for the protection of the child or children concerned. Such protection extends to its physical, educational, moral and mental welfare. Save only to that small extent, a health authority does not have a policing role in society. So where the confidence of, for example, HIV infection is respected by the health authority and not communicated to the patient's sexual partner, the law will not make the health authority liable to that partner who subsequently develops AIDS. No duty of care is owed to such an adult but the position may be different if the person at risk is a child. The ability for patients to seek help and counselling without fear of publication of their innermost secrets is of compelling public importance.

American courts have apparently taken a different view of the responsibilities of medical practitioners: *Tarasoff v. Regents of University of California* (1976) is a case of non-disclosure where a psychiatrist was sued by a person injured by his patient. The court held he had failed to exercise reasonable care to protect the injured party from danger.

The courts will not assist a dissatisfied patient whose confidence has been breached where in the opinion of the court there is an important public interest element justifying that breach. In the case of *W v. Egdell*

((1992) WLR 471) the Court of Appeal refused to assist a psychopath whose discharge from custody was thwarted when the defendant psychiatrist sent a confidential report on him to the Home Office to demonstrate that his release was prejudicial to the safety of the public.

No clear guidelines have yet been given by any medical professional organisation as to the recommended response of a medical worker who faces a 'dilemma' between the public interest in maintaining confidence balanced against the public interest to protect others. There is no dilemma in the case of children – the child's interests are paramount. The existence of a duty of care by members of the medical profession to the public would impose on the profession a potential liability of almost unlimited scope. The judiciary have attempted to discourage the medical profession from practising defensively and I see no drift by the courts to widen the legal responsibility of the medical profession to members of the public.

Conclusion: A new accountability?

Geoffrey Hunt

The democratic process

Some of the contributors to this volume may disagree with my understanding of whistleblowing in the account I give in this conclusion and
in my introduction. No consensus was established between us about its
meaning before the collection was put together and certainly readers
should not ascribe my views to anyone else.

I have spoken to people who see it as 'media hype' and others who
think in terms of isolated incidents. Certainly, on occasion an act of
whistleblowing is a one-off occurrence which in no way reflects upon
the institution as a whole or in part. Sometimes, however, it reflects
upon the inadequacy of a quite local practice or procedure or policy, or
absence of such. Much more important and disturbing for all of us is
whistleblowing as a symptom of a *general lack of institutional accountability*. In this situation whistleblowing is rather like steam escaping
from a boiler under excessive pressure.

I think all the evidence indicates that it is the last situation which now
obtains in the health service, and probably elsewhere in our public sector institutions such as the social services, the civil service and local
government. There are some predisposing factors (as David Pilgrim
pointed out) which predate the market reforms in health care delivery;
certainly hierarchical structures had become ossified and out of keeping
with developments in delivery such as multidisciplinary team work, new
technology and new conceptions of illness and health. However, it now
appears that for every whistleblowing case which the media highlights
there are dozens of cases of staff who raise a concern and then drop it
when they understand what they are up against. For every case of a
dropped concern there are thousands of staff who are aware of substandard practice, patient neglect and abuse, and inadequate procedures,
practices and policies but who feel powerless to voice any concern.
Frank discussions I have had with groups of nurses all over the UK in
the last few years confirm this on the whole.

It may be thought that we are dealing with two separate issues here: questions of standards of practice and care, and questions of the accountability of the health services. The prevailing official ideology links the two through the notion of consumer choice. The belief is that a free market in health care will raise quality in the same way in which a free market in computers or videos raises the value for money of those goods. In this ideology the market is supposed to carry out the function of the political process. People express their choices through their purchasing power rather than through political, social and institutional means. And, since government is supposedly 'minimal' in any case, there is no great need to worry about public accountability in any except the accounting or financial audit sense.

This is not the place to consider this in any detail, but it needs to be said that in reality there is no free market in health care in the UK even if some separate elements of a market system are grafted on in a clumsy and largely unworkable fashion. The neglect and undermining of the *democratic process* of public accountability in the health service (as elsewhere in the public sector) has been disastrous for standards of care and practice. The market has not performed the task and cannot do so.

A dozen ways to shoot the messenger

While one should try to be positive about the subject of accountability, emphasising what is necessary for good practice in management and health care (see below), it is judicious perhaps for the conscientious employee about to raise a concern to be aware of what they might expect in the worst scenario. While one hopes and works for the best, one needs all along be prepared for the worst. Just as the citizen at large has lost touch with the realities of democratic decay in the UK, so the health service employee is often (even now) quite unsuspecting about the degree and scale of defensive, capricious or ignorant behaviour on the part of those entrusted with authority.

Furthermore, it is a worthwhile exercise when thinking about reforms to ask why institutions respond in the specific non-accountable ways that they sometimes do. A brief overview of the institutional alternatives to accountable practice would be amusing if they were not so tragic for the victims. One could roughly arrange these by the degree of defensiveness to which the authority feels driven.

Hot air

The authorities will appear at first to share one's concern. Many words will be generated, insubstantial memoranda may fly about, a meeting may be convened, and promises will be made. No action will be taken, except perhaps the most trivial. At a later date any conversation not recorded on paper may be strenuously denied.

Send to Coventry

A change of mood comes over certain managers and colleagues. Initially this is quite subtle. Greetings, smiles and friendly banter are less frequent. At first you brush it off. Then it becomes more pronounced. Eyebrows are raised mysteriously, you are avoided and left out of events and decisions, sarcastic comments are made. If you mention it you may find that your mental health is questioned.

Close ranks

It is clear that what you said to one colleague or manager has been passed on, and possibly distorted, to his or her peers. When you approach a manager further up the line it is clear that they have been forewarned. Your concern has somehow created an anti-you group. You are identified as a 'trouble-maker' by most people with any authority, and any attempt to raise your concern is now preempted and prejudged. Some of your colleagues feel that your complaint demeans them by implication.

Stonewall

When you raise your concerns formally you find that your letters are unanswered, the manager is never available, promises to 'get back to you' are broken, you are passed on to someone who eventually sends you a letter saying something like 'your concern has been investigated, nothing is amiss, and the matter is now closed'. You may be told directly not to send any more memos or letters.

Biomedical diagnosis

It is suggested that you have been under a 'lot of stress lately' and that you ought to visit the occupational health department, a counsellor or your GP. You are asked if you are 'coping'. It emerges, unknown to you, that you have been informally diagnosed as anxious, depressed, paranoid, having a personality disorder, or as being 'neurotic', too old or too fat.

Spying

A colleague is passing on information about you (and has, perhaps, been asked to do so). You are the object of close observation, fault-finding, and perhaps your mail is being opened and your telephone bugged. Some of your work goes wrong or astray and you wonder about sabotage. If you mention this it is taken as further evidence that you are unable to cope or 'paranoid'.

Grind down

Work becomes more difficult. Your workload increases, you get the tough end of the rota, you are transferred to the most difficult work area, demotion looks more probable than promotion, you do not get your holidays when you want, you are asked to share an office or move out of the one you have, your phone line is put on 'internal calls only' or taken away.

Sticks and carrots

An intermediary, usually a union official, will call you aside for 'a chat' in which offers are made to you concerning promotion, a generous severance package or some other benefit. These will be linked in coded terminology with your concern – the suggestion being that you drop it in return for the benefit. Alternatively, or if you refuse to accept the carrot, veiled threats will be made such as 'Are you sure you wouldn't be happier working elsewhere?'. These become overt threats such as 'You are jeopardising your future' and 'You won't be working here much longer'. If you raised concerns about colleagues, such as their abuse of patients, you may find that you receive hate mail and threats of violence.

Character assassination

Aspersions will be cast on your character, your personal conduct, your personal past, your political views, your class or ethnic origin, or your sexual orientation. These may progress to accusations of abuse of clients, theft of documents, lying, disloyalty, breach of confidentiality, and the like.

First strike

Official countercomplaints may be formulated against you in a disciplinary hearing before your own concerns are addressed or instead of addressing them. You may be made a scapegoat. Disciplinary or grievance procedures may be used as a preemptive or retaliatory measure. The authorities will attempt to get their revenge in first.

Make redundant

Your presence is no longer tolerable. You may be suspended and then dismissed or there may be a reorganisation in which your post is made redundant. You will proceed to an industrial tribunal. If you win you are paid a maximum of £11 000 – which the authorities consider cheap at the price.

Cosmetic reshuffle

If your concerns were of a serious nature, especially if an inquiry took place, then there will be some changes at your workplace of a cosmetic nature. Some posts may be reshuffled, but it is unlikely that policies will be revised or that managerial heads will roll. Certainly no acknowledgement will be made that there is any connection between your raising a concern and the changes which followed.

Possible reforms

What is necessary for the democratic renewal of the health and other public sector services? What should go into a new accountability? Fragments of a programme of reform appear in this book, and I conclude by attempting to bring these together in bold outline form.

- A culture of concern
- A bill of rights
- Freedom of information
- Separation of powers
- Participative decision making
- Standards of care framework
- Coherent complaints system
- Health standards inspectorate
- Ethical health care professionals
- Ethical management
- Ethical audit
- Reform of law of confidence
- Recognition of duty to disclose

- Reform of employment law
- Whistleblower protection legislation

A culture of concern

While I certainly do not believe that *everything* has to change before *anything* changes, no change will really be of lasting significance if it does not play its part in bringing about a overall change in workplace culture. In a genuine workplace *community* there should be a general receptivity to any concern raised. A concern raised by one employee ought to be received by everyone in the workplace as 'our' concern. In this way a concern is shared and the means to addressing the concern are collectively identified and acted upon. In this environment no one would dream of channelling their concern through a grievance or complaints procedure.

Bill of rights

A modern constitution with a bill of rights embodying freedom of speech would go a long way towards generating the background for a culture of concern. It would give all employees a sense that speaking up is not anti-social but recognised and defended by the State itself. It would help overcome the divide between one's role as citizen and one's role as an employee. To be a conscientious employee is at the same time to be a good citizen.

Freedom of information

Legislation to guarantee freedom of information would bring the UK in line with other democracies. It would give the public access to a panoply of government information, furthering open and democratic government and recognising the citizen's right to know what is being done with public money and how and why. In addition, there is a need for greater public access to official meetings and for the official recognition of, and support for, the independent and grass-roots generation and use of information.

Separation of powers

This principle ought to be respected through the institution of appropriate procedures, rules and sanctions at all levels in the health and other public services in order to avoid conflicts of interests which work against the public good. For example, the role of purchasers must be separated from that of suppliers, executive powers in health care delivery separated from commercial interests, disciplinary powers from the managerial role, and political powers from managerial and administrative roles. A right of independent appeal should be recognised at all levels of employment. Consideration might be given to an NHS Tribunal or to strengthening the powers of the Health Commissioner in dealing with staff concerns.

Participative decision making

The making of decisions affecting the public must be opened up at all levels to the public through mechanisms of election and direct represen-tation, consultation, access to public meetings, decentralisation, and the empowerment of Community Health Councils to investigate and moni-tor at all levels. In particular health authorities should have elected rep-resentatives. Quangos are undemocratic and dangerous and should be abolished.

Standards of care framework

A national and comprehensive standards of care framework should be set through a consensual process of consultation involving major input from the public, patients' groups, consumer organisations, nurses, health visitors, midwives, doctors and other professional health carers. Enforceable safeguards to protect these standards will be necessary.

Coherent complaints system

In a culture of concern complaints will be minimal. However, if com-plaints need to be made then they should be addressed in a spirit of open-ness and cooperation. To this end staff complaints and patient complaints should be brought together in a single coherent and independent system. This might be supported by a funded system of patient advocacy.

Health standards inspectorate

The statutory bodies which regulate the health care professions need to be reformed and brought together in one coherent inspectorate with the same rules for all professional groups – nurses, doctors, physiothera-pists, osteopaths, health care assistants, etc. Such an inspectorate must be publicly accountable through mechanisms of representation and must adhere strictly to principles of natural justice, due process and openness.

Ethical health care professionals

There is a need for a new kind of professional, one who adheres to an ethics of openness and partnership with clients rather than an ethics of closure, defensiveness and 'reputation' (Hunt, 1994). Such a professional will act as patient advocate and will take their responsibilities beyond the one-to-one client relationship to a wider *social* obligation. Some indication of this new professional attitude is given by sections of the American Nurses' Association Code for Nurses, which it may be appropriate to adopt in the UK codes for health carers:

10. The nurse participates in the profession's effort to protect the public from misinformation and misrepresentation and to maintain the integrity of nursing.
11. The nurse collaborates with members of the health professions and other citizens in promoting community and national efforts to meet the health needs of the public.

(Benjamin and Curtis 1986, p. 181)

Ethical management

Most urgent of all perhaps, management needs to undergo a significant cultural change. The current problems go far beyond those of some 'bad apples'. Managers need to be open, non-defensive team workers who are well-informed about shop floor difficulties and who understand *their* duty of loyalty to employees and the public. Managers should be regulated, subject to a professional code of conduct and disciplinable in a publicly accountable fashion.

Ethical audit

An audit of the adequacy and efficacy of all those procedures, rules, mechanisms and tacit understandings which maintain the public accountability of managers and employees must take place regularly in any health care institution in an open and free manner with provision for reform.

Law of confidence

The appropriate bodies should provide clear guidance on the law of confidence. In particular, guidance is needed on *what* is confidential and on the distinction between, on the one hand, the professional observance of confidentiality to protect patients/clients from harm and respect their autonomy and, on the other hand, commercial confidentiality or trade secrecy. The abuse of the principle of confidentiality to gag conscientious employees should cease. In any case, it needs to be recognised that most gagging clauses in employment contracts as well as gagging severance contracts are couched in such general terms as to be unenforceable.

I suggest, for discussion, that a health care employer's appeal to 'confidentiality' to silence a professional health carer is *inter alia* unjustifiable when:

1. The professional would by complying infringe the rule of professional ethics that the clients' interests are paramount.
2. The professional would by complying infringe the duty to share information with another professional on a need-to-know basis for the adequate treatment and care of patients.
3. The professional would by complying infringe the rule of professional ethics that, having exhausted internal channels for expressing concern or complaint, they have a duty to disclose in the public interest.
4. Something is deemed to be confidential *solely* in respect of it having been stipulated to be so by an authority.
5. The *sole* or principal ground for non-disclosure is the administrative inconvenience or managerial embarrassment or supposed institutional damage which would or might result from disclosure.

Duty to disclose

Generally, we all need to assume that information may be disclosed unless a good reason can be provided for non-disclosure rather than the current widespread assumption that information is to be kept secret unless a good reason can be provided for disclosing it. The burden of proof should be put on the employer to prove that information should be protected. Consideration should be given to codifying a professional duty to disclose (and, therefore, in what ways non-disclosure may be an offence).

Reform of employment law

The law should be amended to discourage the dismissal of staff for causing embarrassment by raising concerns in the public interest and to provide remedy to those so dismissed. An employee who is shown to have been dismissed for raising a public concern should, perhaps, receive double compensation. There should be a general legal provision that professionals who are subject to statutory bodies should have their code of conduct incorporated in their contract of employment. Industrial tribunals also need reform to take special cognisance of the circumstances and needs of whistleblowers.

Whistleblower legislation

Consideration should be given to the merits and disadvantages of legislation specifically designed to protect the whistleblower. Such legislation might serve to protect whistleblowers from intimidation and victimisation, and provide for compensation. It might even go as far as offering rewards along the lines of the American False Claims Act which allows individuals who blow the whistle on fraud in government contracts to collect as a reward a portion of any money recovered for the taxpayer.

The case of Graham Pink

I close this book, as I opened it, with the words of John Hendy QC, the barrister who defended Graham Pink, the courageous charge nurse, who lost his job when he stood up for decent patient care in his hospital in Stockport. In that case the nurses' regulatory body (the UKCC) would not accept that there was a case for Mr Pink being disciplined for breach of confidentiality. In the event this did not help Mr Pink very much, since the employer sacked him for a supposed breach anyway. The UKCC, and other regulatory bodies, do not appear to carry much weight with employers, who often ignore them at will. Unfortunately, the UKCC refused to proceed against the nurse managers whom Mr Pink claimed had failed in their duty to act on his concerns about standards of care, and refused to provide a reason for not proceeding.

After spending a great deal of public money defending the indefensible the health authority conceded that Mr Pink had been unfairly dismissed. John Hendy QC, then stated:

> The evidence revealed by cross examination in the first two weeks of the Tribunal showed that the alleged main ground for Mr Pink's dismissal was that he was responsible for an article in the local paper in July 1990 highlighting lack of staffing. This, it was alleged, constituted breach of patient confidentiality. But the evidence showed that by then nothing had been done about staffing levels and the investigations into it were kept secret from Mr Pink. By then he had pursued every other possible avenue open to

him including writing to every level of management right up to the Secretary of State for Health. He was not favoured with any positive response. . . . It is plain that the real reason Mr Pink was sacked was because, having failed to remedy the matter internally, he complained publicly about the lack of nurses. Criticism is something the Health Authority was not prepared to tolerate. So it sacked him. Now, as Mr Pink sees it, to avoid further damaging cross examination it has conceded unfair dismissal. . . . This case has vindicated nurses who, after taking up internally failures to provide adequate patient care, raise such issues publicly. The evidence confirmed that the standard form Health Authority contract of employment with Mr Pink incorporated the UKCC's standards. These make clear that nurses (who have their own professional autonomy) in the last resort must each decide when the public interest requires that they speak out: it is a matter for them and they cannot be gagged by their employers.

(Hendy, 1993)

References

BENJAMIN, M. AND CURTIS, J. (1986) *Ethics in Nursing.* Oxford University Press, Oxford.

HENDY, J. (1993) Press Statement following Graham Pink's Industrial Tribunal, Lincoln's Inn, London.

HUNT, G. (1994) New Professionals? New Ethics? In *Expanding the Role of the Nurse*, G. Hunt and P. Wainwright (eds). Blackwell Scientific, Oxford.

Index